History of Medicine

The enthralling saga of man's struggle against disease

**As per MCI Guidelines on the Foundation Course for the
Undergraduate Medical Education Program, 2019—Orientation Module**

"You have to know the past to understand the present."
—American scientist Carl Sagan (1934–96)

History of Medicine

The enthralling saga of man's struggle against disease

As per MCI Guidelines on the Foundation Course for the
Undergraduate Medical Education Program, 2019—Orientation Module

Suyog Sindhu

MBBS, MD (Pharmacology)

Assistant Professor
Department of Pharmacology
King George's Medical University
Lucknow
UP

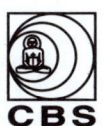

CBS Publishers and Distributors Pvt Ltd

New Delhi • Bengaluru • Chennai • Kochi • Kolkata • Mumbai
Bhopal • Bhubaneswar • Hyderabad • Jharkhand • Nagpur • Patna
• Pune • Uttarakhand • Dhaka (Bangladesh) • Kathmandu (Nepal)

History of Medicine

The enthralling saga of man's struggle against disease

ISBN: 978-93-89565-75-1

Copyright © Author and Publisher

First Edition: 2020

Published by Satish Kumar Jain and produced by Varun Jain for

CBS Publishers & Distributors Pvt Ltd

4819/XI Prahlad Street, 24 Ansari Road, Daryaganj, New Delhi 110 002, India.
Ph: 23289259, 23266861, 23266867   Website: www.cbspd.com
Fax: 011-23243014   e-mail: delhi@cbspd.com; cbspubs@airtelmail.in.
Corporate Office: 204 FIE, Industrial Area, Patparganj, Delhi 110 092
Ph: 011-4934 4934   Fax: 011-4934 4935   e-mail: publishing@cbspd.com;
publicity@cbspd.com

Branches

- **Bengaluru:** Seema House 2975, 17th Cross, K.R. Road,
  Banasankari 2nd Stage, Bengaluru 560 070, Karnataka
  Ph: +91-80-26771678/79   Fax: +91-80-26771680   e-mail: bangalore@cbspd.com
- **Chennai:** 7, Subbaraya Street, Shenoy Nagar, Chennai 600 030, Tamil Nadu
  Ph: +91-44-26680620, 26681266   Fax: +91-44-42032115   e-mail: chennai@cbspd.com
- **Kochi:** 68/1534, 35, 36 Power House Road, Opp. KSEB, Kochi 682018, Kerala
  Ph: +91-484-4059061-65   Fax: +91-484-4059065   e-mail: kochi@cbspd.com
- **Kolkata:** 6/B, Ground Floor, Rameswar Shaw Road, Kolkata-700 014, West Bengal
  Ph: +91-33-22891126, 22891127, 22891128 e-mail: kolkata@cbspd.com
- **Mumbai:** 83-C, Dr E Moses Road, Worli, Mumbai-400018, Maharashtra
  Ph: +91-22-24902340/41   Fax: +91-22-24902342   e-mail: mumbai@cbspd.com

Representatives

• Bhopal	0-8319310552	• Bhubaneswar	0-9911037372	• Hyderabad	0-9885175004
• Jharkhand	0-9811541605	• Nagpur	0-9421945513	• Patna	0-9334159340
• Pune	0-9623451994	• Uttarakhand	0-9716462459	• Dhaka	01912-003485
• Kathmandu	977-9818742655			(Bangladesh)	
(Nepal)					

Printed at : **India Binding House, Noida, UP, India.**

to

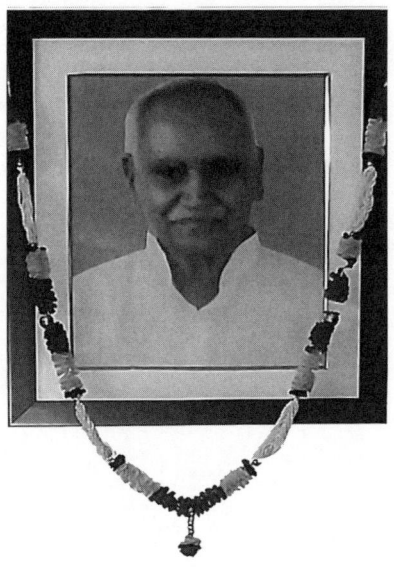

my affectionate father-in-law, late Sri Harikant Dwivedi,
who always encouraged my work when he was alive,
and whose blessings from his heavenly abode keep me going

Foreword

History of Medicine: *Enthralling saga of man's struggle against disease* has an essence of its own, both in scope and content. It is different from many existing books on the history of medicine. It does justice in highlighting the key milestones in the development of medicine. Its coverage stretches from prehistoric times to modern times. The presentation is simple yet interesting. This enables one to understand and comprehend the evolution of medicine better. Learning of history in way of a saga will preserve the rich heritage of medicine.

It gives me immense pleasure to declare that the author has made all efforts to meet the need of all the medical students. Recently Competency Based Curriculum for the Undergraduate Medical Education has been introduced. The foundation module of this curriculum includes the history of medicine as a pivotal and integral part. I am sure that this book would be useful for undergraduate medical students.

Dr Harmeet Singh Rehan
Director-Professor and Head
Department of Pharmacology
Lady Hardinge Medical College
New Delhi

Preface

As a teacher, I have always felt a strong obligation to teach my students about the evolution of 'medicine' and 'doctors'. The result is in the form of this book. The purpose of this book is to enlighten the budding doctors about their roots. 'Medicine' and 'doctors' as we see today have emerged after a continuous journey of innumerable years. This book takes the readers in wonderland of early doctors in the form of 'Shamans'. One meets Hippocrates, Galen, Paracelsus, and many more fascinating personalities from the past. The saga ends with the living legends from India.

The story of the evolution of medicine stretches from prehistoric times to modern times. It is so vast that no book can cover it entirely. Sir William Osler had once remarked, "the value of experience is not in seeing much but seeing in wisely." In no way is this book a complete treatise of the vast history of medicine. It is a key-hole to the endless world of inventions and discoveries in the field of medicine.

I hope this book will make an enjoyable reading. Suggestions for improvements from teachers and students are most welcome.

Suyog Sindhu

Acknowledgements

It is an emotional moment to thank all my teachers who gave me formal training in medicine. Heartfelt thanks to Dr IP Jain, Dr SP Singh and late Dr Suresh Singh who enlightened me during my postgraduation at GSVM Medical College, Kanpur.

I find no words to express my indebtedness to Dr VK Verma. I feel blessed to have his words of wisdom everytime I am in confused state of mind. Dr Hemant K Singh, in spite of his busy schedule, has always acted as my guiding light.

It would be injustice if I do not name people who always support me as pillars—Dr Priyanka Singh, Dr Sujeet Gautum, Dr Puja Khanna, Dr Rashmi Singh, Dr Neeraj Aggrawal, Dr Niranjan K Singh, Dr Amit Chaudhary and Dr Savita Chaudhary.

I take this opportunity to thank Mr YN Arjuna, Senior Vice President—Publishing, Editorial and Publicity, and his team for editing and publishing my book.

As a token of appreciation, I thank my spouse, Dr Reetesh Dwivedi, and my kids, Devang and Divit, for allowing me time to write this book.

Suyog Sindhu

Contents

Dawn of Medicine

Somewhere around 6500 BC.

Everything was fine. Five men clad in animal skins around loin walked through long grass, looking for food. One of them was feeling weak and uneasy to follow his companions for the hunt. Unwillingly he drudged behind while his fellow mates boisterously searched for food (Fig. 1). "Shhh! look there. A pair of dodos." All men instantly dived their heads inside the grass and hastily made their way towards the hunt. "Thunk! Thunk! Thunk! Thunk! Thunk!" Amidst the sound of arrows being shot towards the target, emerged an unexpected loud shriek. The drudging man fell on the ground with a thud. Others watched him helplessly as his

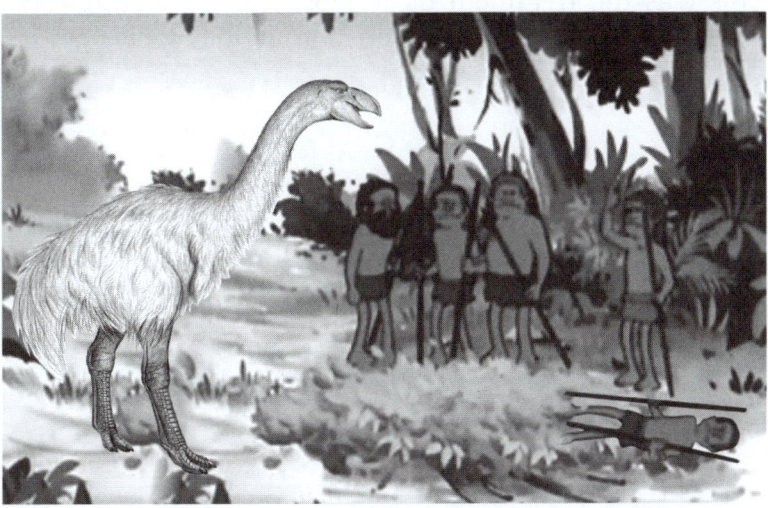

Fig. 1: One of the prehistoric hunters fallen on ground while his fellow mates hunting a dodo

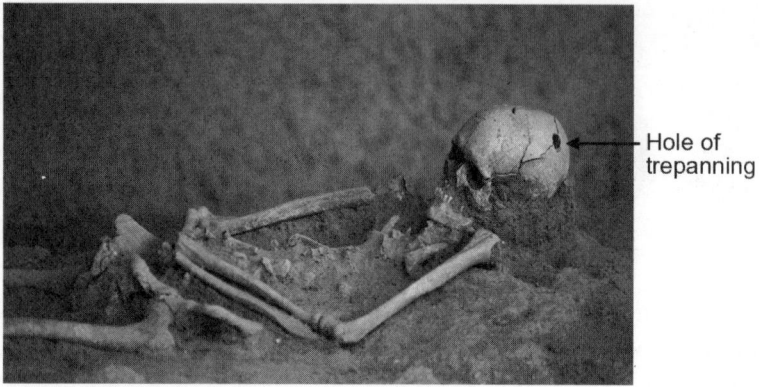

Hole of
trepanning

Fig. 2: Evidence of trepanning from prehistoric times

body went into jerks and his mouth frothed. They helped him back to their native cave once he revived back.

Later that evening, the clan of prehistoric men gathered to enjoy the food that they had collected that day. After the feast was over, the man whose body had undergone abnormal movements was laid on the ground. One old, wise member of the clan meticulously drilled a hole in his head using his instruments of flintstone and bowstring (Fig. 2). This was the treatment of epilepsy by trepanning (also known as trephining or trephination) in the Stone Age!

Medicine in Early Civilizations

Medicine developed at an early stage in Egypt, India and China. The earliest Indian and Chinese medical texts that we possess are decidedly younger than those of Egypt. While Egyptian medicine completed its course long ago, ancient Indian and Chinese medicines are still fully alive and are practiced by millions of people even today. At the end of this chapter, it would be remarked that in each of these archaic practices of medicine the common purpose is to "protect the health of the healthy and pacify the disease of the diseased".

EGYPT

The medicine of ancient Egypt shaped ideas of the civilizations around it, including the medicine of Greek and Roman civilizations.

Ancient Egyptians had a widespread reputation for their medical knowledge.

Each of the physicians of Egypt was a specialist committed to one particular branch of medicine. The foundation of medical science was established in Egypt more than fifty centuries ago as evidenced by a mass of documentary evidence, medical 'Papyri'.

Following is a list of the surviving papyri and their locations.

1. The *Ebers Papyrus* preserved at the University of Leipzig, Germany. It is the longest and most famous among all papyri. Written in 1570–1320 BC or even earlier, it deals with diseases of the stomach, action of the heart and its

vessels and surgical treatment of cysts, boils, carbuncles and similar conditions.

2. The *Hearst Papyrus* kept at the University of California. Its contents are similar to those of the Ebers Papyrus.

3. The *Edwin Smith Papyrus* is in the possession of the Historical Society of New York. It comprises medico-magical incantation and prescriptions dealing with the surgical treatment of wounds and fractures.

4. The *Chester Beatty Papyrus*, at the British Museum, contains a series of prescriptions and remedies for diseases of the anus and rectum.

5. The *Berlin Medical Papyrus*, kept at the Berlin Museum, dates back to 1320–1200 BC. It is similar in character to the Ebers and Hearst papyri.

6. The *Kahun Papyrus*, 1991–1786 BC. It deals only with gynecology.

7. The *London Medical Papyrus*, is preserved at the British Museum. It is entirely medico-magical in its contents.

8. A number of medico-magical papyri exist in museums in Paris, Leiden, Turin, Berlin, Budapest, Copenhagen, and Rome.

According to the *Kahun papyri*, it was determined whether a woman would or would not be able to bear children by keeping a bulb of onion or garlic in her vagina over night until dawn. If the specific odor of either appeared in her mouth, she would be able to bear children. The scientific foundation of this fertility test is that onion and garlic contain volatile oils which pass from the cervix through the uterus to the fallopian tubes and, if these are unobstructed, reach the peritoneal cavity which has a very high absorbency to circulation. The route of excretion of these volatile oils is the respiratory tract.

The first specialized hospitals for antenatal care were established in Egypt 4000 years ago. A separate room called *Mamezewas* was built in the house garden or upper story to isolate the mother for two weeks after giving birth and to protect her from puerperal sepsis.

The ancient Egyptians practiced family planning. For example, contraceptive devices of different shapes and sizes were inserted into the uterus. They believed that semen was formed in a man's heart and stored in the holy bone called the sacrum. They said, "he gave her some of his heart" and called the role of man in pregnancy the "beautiful role". There is a temple wall showing a sperm beside an ovum, then the division of a fertilized ovum into two, then four cells!

Topical anesthesia was necessarily practised for minor operations. By putting vinegar (acetic acid) in a certain concentration over marble stone, a cooling effect of carbon dioxide resulted from the interaction with acetic acid. The marble stone thus had an anesthetizing effect!

Trephining, the process of perforating the skull with a surgical instrument was common surgical practice. Skulls of mummies with well-healed edges indicate that patients lived after a trephine operation. This operation required great skill in not injuring the dura mater (covering of the brain), which otherwise would result in exposure of the brain and be fatal. The instruments used for trephinations were hammers, chisels and scraper!

The ancient Egyptians practiced venesection or bloodletting (Fig. 3). Earlier as well as today physicians use this procedure to treat scorpion stings or snakebites.

Egyptian orthopedicians used wooden splints padded with linen and imru, which seems to resemble plaster of Paris.

One of the techniques mentions soaking linen with egg white, wrapping it around the fractured limb after its reduction, and then leaving it to dry.

There were superb techniques in the field of dentistry as well. They used the cavity of a recently extracted tooth or prepared a cavity in the jawbone, then placed a healthy tooth inside the cavity and fixed it to an adjacent tooth using a fine gold wire. They had learnt that the transplant was not rejected if the tooth came from a twin but might be rejected if the tooth came from a person unrelated to the family of the patient.

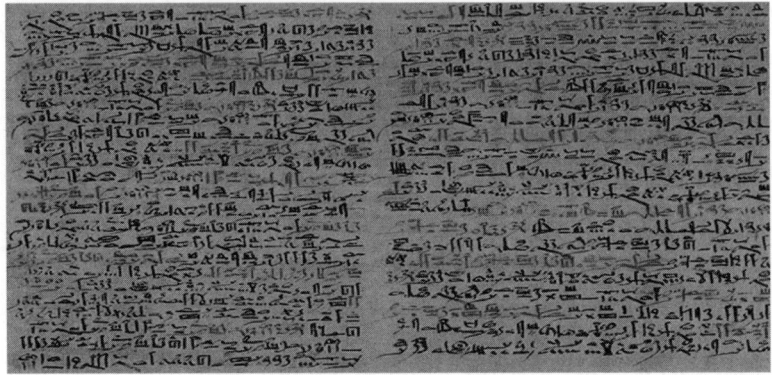

Fig. 3: Ancient Egyptian papyri

The ancient Egyptians brilliantly defined pulse as "speech of the heart through peripheral vessels" and heart as the central organ of the body, essential to both the living and the dead. They theorized that all senses report directly to the heart and that it was the seat of thought, emotion, and intelligence. It was just that they used the term heart equivalent to present day "brain"!

The Egyptians knew about night blindness and treated it with roasted ox liver. As established by modern medicine, ox liver is very rich in vitamin A, and a deficiency of vitamin A causes night blindness!

These are just few examples to make us believe that ancient Egyptians were highly gifted people with great advancements in medical field.

CHINA

Traditional Chinese Medicine (TCM) is an integral part of ancient Chinese civilization. Diagnosis is based on observing, listening or smelling, questioning, touching, knowing the family, family's history and food likes-dislikes. Treatment is based on knowledge acquired through long-term medical practice in combination with an assessment of natural conditions including climate, geography and phenology (the study of periodic effects on plant and animal life cycles influenced by seasonal variations).

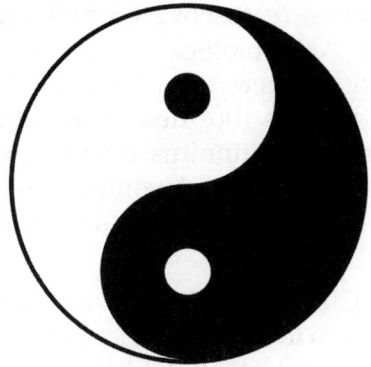

Fig. 4: Yin–Yang

TCM is based on two opposite principals—yin and yang and their interdependence (Fig. 4). These two opposites are in constant motion, creating a fluctuating balance in the healthy body. Disease results when either yin or yang is in a stage of prolonged excess or deficiency.

Through a long evolutionary process, knowledge and experience developed, prescriptions for fighting diseases were accumulated and enriched. The use of fire improved hygiene and health care. The change from raw to cooked food, combined with being able to keep warm, greatly reduced the incidence of disease in Chinese civilization. Use of earthenware appeared during the Neolithic age (5000–3000 BC) and that of elaborately carved stone knives by early Paleolithic age. By the Neolithic age, the knife evolved into a stone needle. As early as 3000 years ago, bronze metallurgy enabled people to make bronze needles. About 2470 years ago, the Iron Age began and iron needles came into use. Needles in different dimensions, lengths, calibers, and shapes with round, blunt or sharp ends are still employed by Chinese physicians for treatment using art of acupuncture and moxibustion (the burning of moxa herb on or near a person's skin as a counterirritant).

There is also an ancient tradition for herbal medicine in China. In prehistoric times, people ate plants, fruits from trees and grasses, worms, and clams (a marine bivalve mollusc with shells of equal size). Later on herbs with medicinal values were discovered and used for treating diseases (Fig. 5). Archeological investigations have found inscriptions and characters on bones and tortoise shells dealing with diseases like headache, abdominal pain, dizziness, common cold, tinnitus, deafness, eye disease, and ulcers, as well as children's and women's diseases and dental diseases such as caries. They also included infectious diseases and parasitosis.

In one of the Chinese medical literature it is mentioned "diseases can be seen in all seasons, for example, head disease in spring, scabies and other itching diseases in summer, malaria and cold diseases in autumn, and asthmatic and coughing diseases in winter"—this indicates the recognition of relationships between seasons and diseases by ancient Chinese.

Ancient Chinese were staunch believers of ethics in medical practice. The general principles for medical morality in TCM were set out in the form of Codex. It includes chapters on medical ethics.

Medical ethics in TCM can be summarized as follows:

1. Be assiduous and love the profession. If you want to become an excellent doctor, you must read extensively to increase your medical knowledge. Ignorant and idle people without aspiration are not qualified to be doctors. Even a doctor with a great deal of knowledge should continuously improve and update his information and skill.

2. Do your best to save lives regardless of payment and rewards. Doctors of TCM must be humanitarians, making no distinction between the rich and the poor.

3. Work in a proper style. A doctor must treat all patients. He must visit them at their homes instead of waiting for patients to come to him. If he does not behave well, or if he has some immodest evil thoughts, he will suffer material and spiritual harm.

4. Adhere to science and fight against superstition. Medicine in China, was intermingled with witchcraft to

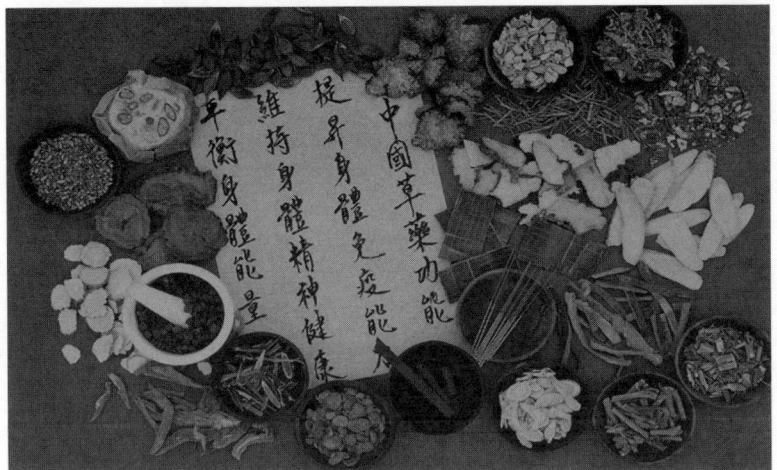

Fig. 5: Use of herbs in traditional Chinese Medicine

some extent at an early stage and both were involved in the development of TCM. However, it was soon realised that they were antagonistic to each other and eventually each had its own separate development. It was emphasized that real doctors must get rid of superstitions and insist on scientific behavior.

The above brief note on TCM throws sufficient light on richness and quality of medical practice in Chinese civilization.

INDIA

Archeological and modern genetic evidence suggest that human populations have migrated into the Indian subcontinent since prehistoric times. The knowledge of the medicinal value of plants and other substances and their uses go back to the time of the earliest settlers. Excavations at different sites suggest that medical interventions such as dentistry and trepanation were practiced as early as 7000 BCE in the Indian subcontinent.

Ayurveda is the indigenious system of medicine that developed here over a span of several ages. In Sanskrit, it means science or wisdom (veda) of life. It is a rationale, logical medical science which has survived from antiquity to the present day. Historical roots suggest that it has paved the way for various branches of medicine. Early Greek medicine embraced many concepts originally described in classical Ayurvedic texts dating back thousands of years. Traditional Tibetan and Chinese medicine also have roots in Ayurveda.

There is collection of anatomical data from ancient India. During the practice of Vedic sacrifice, the anatomy of the sacrificised animal was carefully studied. A crude form of the human body dissection to acquire anatomical knowledge was probably practiced in early times but later the study of anatomy became less important for pattern of medicine followed here.

The idea central to Ayurveda is that "five great elements" earth, water, fire, air and space-make up the entire phenomenal world including the human body. Further a whole system of dietary recommendations forms framework for diagnosis, therapy and treatment in this traditional medicine. It comprises recommendations ranging from preparation and consumption of food, to healthy routines for day and night, sexual life, and rules for ethical conduct. For example, in dietetics it is considered that sweet foods are predominantly made up of the elements earth and water. In the human body fatty tissue is made up mainly of the same elements. This implies that excessive eating of sweet substances increases fatty tissue in the body—this principal goes hand in hand with modern system of medicine! In Ayurvedic practice, the elementary composition of a substance is known by its properties or qualities. The principle is to treat with opposite qualities.

Many Ayurvedic practices predate written records as they were advocated by word of mouth. This body of knowledge is believed to have been originally delivered by God to sages and seers, who were yogis with extraordinary insight, intuition and keen observation of human behavior. They handed down their knowledge to their disciples.

Three ancient books known as the Great Trilogy— *Charaka Samhita, Sushruta Samhita* and *Astanga Hridaya* written in Sanskrit more than 2,000 years ago, are considered the main texts on Ayurvedic medicine. The earliest codified documents are *Charaka Samhita* and *Sushruta Samhita*. *Charak Samhita* deals with internal medicine whereas *Sushruta Samhita* is dominated by surgical procedures. *Sushruta Samhita* discusses nine branches—surgery, ear, nose and throat diseases, toxicology, psychiatry, pediatrics, gynecology, sexology, and virility. It relies on a natural and holistic approach to physical and mental health focusing on interconnections among people, their health, the universe, the body's constitution and life forces. Using these concepts, Ayurvedic physicians prescribe individualized treatments that include herbs, diet, music, massage treatments, exercise and meditation along with lifestyle recommendations.

This traditional Indian medicine identified a wide range ailments including fever, cough, constipation, diarrhea, dropsy, abscesses, seizures, tumours, and leprosy. Treatments included plastic surgery, lithotomy, tonsillectomy, couching (a form of cataract surgery), puncturing to release fluids in the abdomen, extraction of foreign bodies, treatment of anal fistulas, treating fractures, amputations, cesarean sections and stitching of wounds (Fig. 6). The use of herbs and surgical instruments was widespread. Treatments were also prescribed for complex

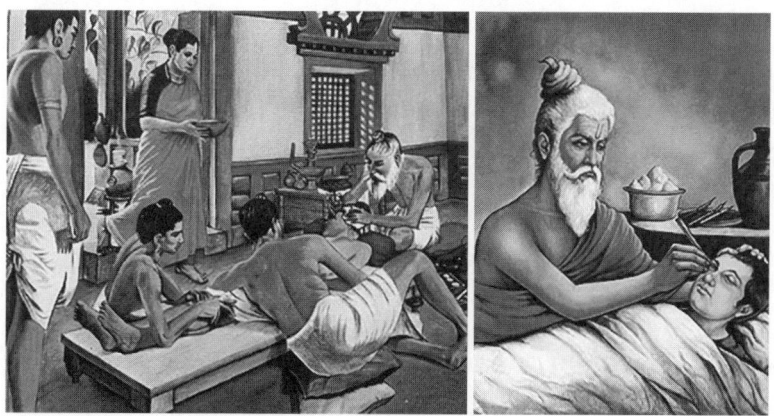

Fig. 6: Cataract surgery by Sushruta

ailments, including angina pectoris, diabetes, hypertension, and stones.

This Indian system of indigenous medicine has regained its importance in present times not only in its country of origin but worldwide!

Timelines in History of Medicine

The history of medicine is long and distinguished one as healers sought to alleviate illness and fix injuries since the dawn of human civilization. It is difficult to spot the starting point of this long journey. The finish point is all the more beyond imagination. As it would be an uphill task to dive into the ocean of history and fish out every stepping stone in path of healing, an attempt has been made in this book to highlight the most remarkable discoveries and discoverers in different timelines of history (Fig. 7).

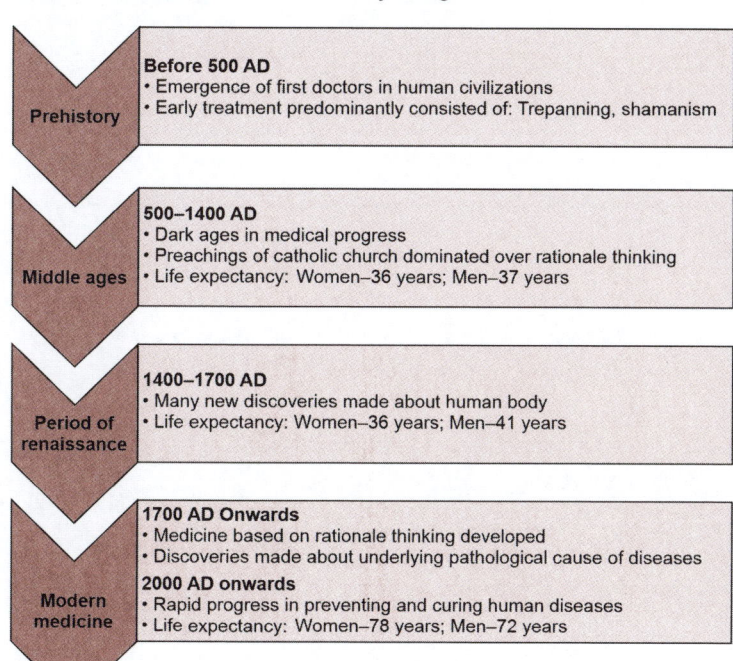

Prehistory

Before 500 AD
• Emergence of first doctors in human civilizations
• Early treatment predominantly consisted of: Trepanning, shamanism

Middle ages

500–1400 AD
• Dark ages in medical progress
• Preachings of catholic church dominated over rationale thinking
• Life expectancy: Women–36 years; Men–37 years

Period of renaissance

1400–1700 AD
• Many new discoveries made about human body
• Life expectancy: Women–36 years; Men–41 years

Modern medicine

1700 AD Onwards
• Medicine based on rationale thinking developed
• Discoveries made about underlying pathological cause of diseases
2000 AD onwards
• Rapid progress in preventing and curing human diseases
• Life expectancy: Women–78 years; Men–72 years

Fig. 7: Different timelines of history

Though there are no fixed points where time can be labelled, history of medicine can be divided in following four timelines in accordance to its advancement. These will be dealt with individually in chapters that follow.

i. Prehistoric medicine (Chapter 4)

ii. Middle Ages (Chapter 5)

iii. Period of Renaissance (Chapter 6)

iv. Modern medicine (Chapter 7)

Prehistoric Medicine
(until 500 BC)

Prehistoric medicine refers to medicine before humans were able to read and write. It covers a vast period, which varies according to regions and cultures. Anthropological and archaeological studies reveal that all cultures during this period of history used a blend of rituals and medical techniques to cure ailments.

Different diseases and ailments were more common in prehistory than today. There is evidence that many people suffered from osteoarthritis, probably caused by the lifting of heavy objects which would have been a daily and necessary task in those times. For example, the transport of latte stones, which involved hyper-extension and torque of the lower back, while dragging the stones, may have contributed to the development of micro fractures in the spine and subsequent spondylolysis. Incidences of cuts, bruises, and breakages of bone, without antiseptics, proper facilities, or knowledge of germs, would become very serious if infected, as they did not have sufficient ways to treat infection. There is also evidence of rickets and osteomalacia (conditions of bone deformity and bone wastage).

The life expectancy in prehistoric times was as low as 25–40 years, with men living longer than women. Archaeological evidence of women and babies found together suggests that many women would have died during the process of childbirth, perhaps accounting for the lower life expectancy in women than men. Also, men as hunters may have sometimes received better food than the woman, who would consequently have been less resistant to disease. Another possible explanation for the shorter life spans of prehistoric humans may be malnutrition.

For early human civilizations to maintain good health, prevent diseases and care for wounds was as important as it is today and this paved path for primitive medicine.

Herbal medicine is the earliest scientific medical practice common to all early human civilizations. In the process of discovering which plants are edible, early humans identified many which could cure ailments or soothe a fever. The early physicians stumbled upon herbal substances of real power, without understanding the manner of their working!

- One classical example is doctors in ancient India gave an extract of foxglove to patients with legs swollen due to dropsy (edema in peripheral parts of body due to congestive heart failure—CHF). In modern medicine digitalis, a constituent of foxglove, is a standard stimulant for the heart in CHF!
- Similarly, curare which was smeared on the tip of arrows in the Amazonian jungles to paralyze the prey thousands of years ago, is an important muscle relaxant in modern surgery!
- The birch polypore fungus, found among the possessions of a mummified man in alpine environments, was used as a laxative by prehistoric peoples living in Northern Europe. Today we know that it brings on short bouts of diarrhoea when ingested!

Anthropological studies reveal that apart from using herbal substances, the primitive physician acted as **Shaman or witch-doctor** whose main duty was to appease or expel the evil spirit troubling the sick person.

Shamans maintained the health of their tribe by gathering and distributing herbs, performing minor surgical procedures, providing medical advice, and supernatural treatments such as charms, spells, and amulets to ward off evil spirits. The protocol of treatment followed by them included performing a ceremony over the patient, attended by family and friends. It consisted of magic formulas, prayers, and drumming. Then, from patients' recalling of their past and possible offenses against their religion or tribal rules, the nature of the disease and how to treat it was decided by the shaman.

Surgical methods were also employed apart from herbs and shamanism by early medicine men. In Europe, in Asia and particularly in Peru, well-preserved mummies having the hole in the skull as result of trepanning (also known as trephining or trephination) have been discovered (Figs 8 and 9). It is not known how such operations were done. One method may be cutting and scraping away at the bone of the skull with a sharp flint, until a hole is virtually rubbed away. Another may be making a circle of small holes with a flint drill and then cutting between them. Reasoning behind trepanning was to cure certain conditions such as headaches and epilepsy which were considered to be effects of an evil spirit trapped within a person.

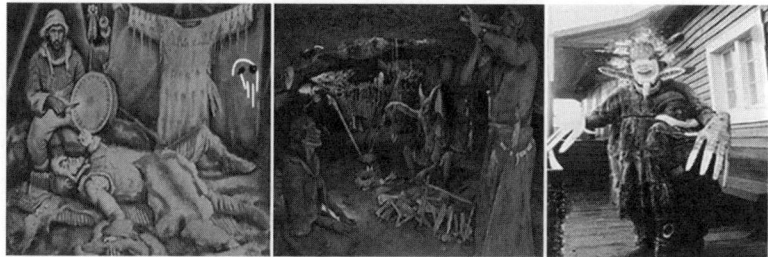

Fig. 8: Shamanism

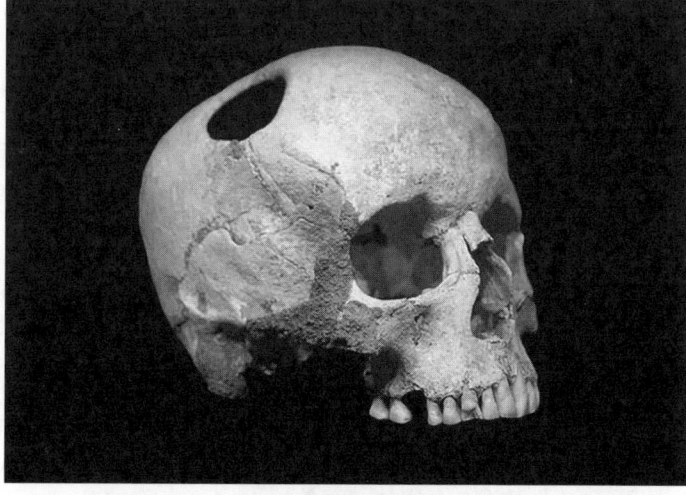

Fig. 9: Trepanning

PROMINENT PHYSICIANS IN PRE-HISTORIC ERA

HIPPOCRATES

Hippocrates was born on the Aegean island of Kos around 460 BC. Little is known about his life experiences. Historians rely on a biography written some 500 years after his death by another Greek physician, Soranus and a collection of medical writings in form of more than 60 medical books commonly called the Hippocratic Corpus.

His formal name was Hippocrates Asclepiades, meaning "descendant of (the doctor-god) Asclepios". He was born in a wealthy family, as son of Praxithea and Heracleides. He learnt medicine from his father and another physician Herodicos. Historians believe Hippocrates traveled throughout the Greek mainland and possibly Libya and Egypt practicing medicine.

Known for his teaching as much as his healing abilities, Hippocrates passed on his medical knowledge to his two sons and started a school for medicine on the island of Kos around 400 BC. It was probably here that many of the methods attributed to Hippocrates were developed.

Much of what is known about these methods comes from Hippocratic Corpus which is considered the oldest

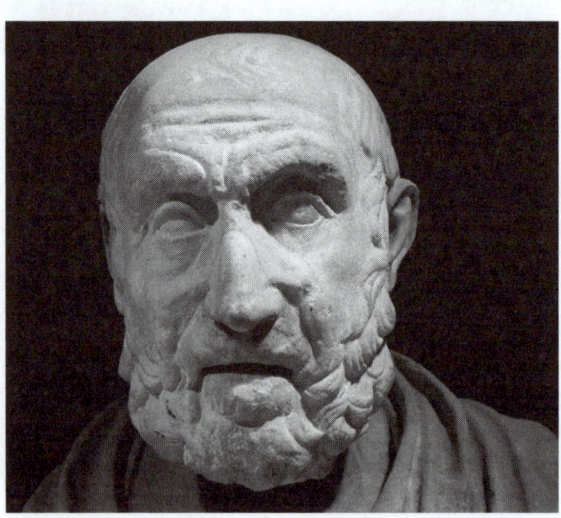

collection of writings on medicine. Compiled 100 years after his death, historians believe the documents may be the work of many different physicians practicing medicine during Hippocrates' lifetime and later. However, a unique aspect of the writings is that they share basic assumptions about how the human body works and the nature of disease. The books were written in reference to different fields of medicine for physicians, pharmacists, and the layperson, not so much to practice medicine, but to be able to talk with the doctor!

According to the Corpus, Hippocratic medicine recommended a healthy diet and physical exercise as a remedy for most ailments. If this did not reduce sickness, some type of medication was recommended. Plants were processed for their medicinal elements. The Corpus also describes how joints could be repositioned, the importance of keeping records of case histories and treatments, and the relationship between the weather and some illnesses.

Though Hippocratic medicine believed disease was caused by natural forces, instead of the will of the gods as was commonly believed, it did not have a firm understanding of the nature of what makes people ill. Doctors at that time only observed sick people not the diseases themselves. Most descriptions of internal organs were based on what could be seen or felt externally. Dissections of animals were performed to make comparisons with the human body as Greek ethics forbid dissection of humans.

The very familiar "Hippocratic Oath" is a document on medical practices, ethics, and morals. Originally, Hippocrates was credited with composing the oath, however, newer research indicates it was written after his death by other physicians influenced by the medical practices in the Corpus. Though not applied in its original form today, the many modernized versions that exist serve as foundation for the oath that medical graduates take at the start of their careers. Some of the basic tenets of the oath include practicing medicine to the best of one's ability, sharing knowledge with other physicians, employing sympathy, compassion and understanding, respecting the privacy of patients and helping to prevent disease whenever possible.

Little is known about Hippocrate's death or his age, though it is widely held that he died in the Ancient Greek town of Larissa, around 377 BC. What is known is that he made a major contribution to medicine and set a standard for ethical practices!

GALEN

Galen was an ancient Greek physician and surgeon in the Roman Empire. He was also a renowned philosopher of his times though most of his philosophical writings have been lost. As a very prominent physician, he greatly influenced the development of various scientific disciplines like anatomy, physiology, pathology and neurology, and was considered an authority on medical theory and practice in Europe until the mid-17th century.

Galen, also known as Aelius Galenus or Claudius Galenus, was born in September 130 AD in the city of Pergamon (modern-day Bergama, Turkey), a major cultural hub in those times. His father, Aelius Nicon, was a prosperous architect and builder with scholarly interests.

He received a good education and his father expected him to undertake a traditional career in philosophy or politics.

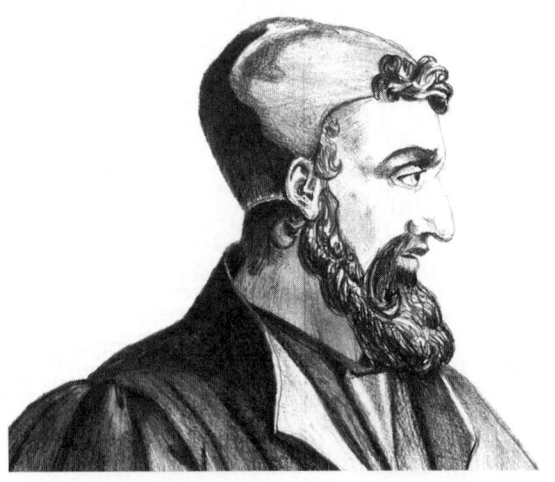

However, one night his father had a dream in which a god commanded him to send Galen to study medicine. Thus Galen started studying medicine at a local sanctuary dedicated to Asclepius, the god of medicine. His understanding of anatomy and medicine was greatly influenced by the theories of ancient Greek physicians such as Hippocrates. He travelled widely, exposing himself to a variety of medical theories and discoveries, and also studied at the great medical school of Alexandria. He eventually embarked on a career as a physician and soon gained prominence with his in-depth medical knowledge and surgical skills.

He returned to his hometown in 157 AD and worked as physician to the gladiators of the High Priest of Asia. This was a prestigious position as the gladiators were among the most influential and wealthy men in Asia. While working in this position, he also furthered his studies in theoretical medicine and philosophy.

He went to Rome in 162 AD and established himself as an efficient physician. However, he was also short-tempered and used to antagonize the less skilled physicians. Because of his temperament he earned himself a considerable number of detractors and when his enmity with other medical practitioners became serious, he fled the city fearing for his safety!

Later when a great plague broke out in Rome in 169 AD, he was summoned back. There he became the physician to Emperor Marcus Aurelius. Even though Aurelius died in 180 AD, Galen remained at the court as a physician to his successor Commodus for much of his life. It was here in court that Galen wrote extensively on medical subjects.

Galen's primary interest was in human anatomy and he considered the study of anatomy to be the foundation of medical knowledge. Since performing dissections on human corpses was forbidden under Roman law, he frequently experimented on such lower animals as apes, pigs, sheep, and goats. He left a physiological model of the human body that became the mainstay of the medieval physician's university anatomy curriculum, but it suffered greatly from stasis and intellectual stagnation because some of Galen's ideas were incorrect as he did not dissect a human body.

He was a skilled surgeon and much ahead of his times. He was known to have performed complicated surgeries on delicate organs like eyes and brains. His works on the circulatory system were also much ahead of his times.

Galen was a prolific writer and is believed to have produced more work than any author in antiquity. It is possible that he might have written up to 600 manuscripts. A major fire destroyed most of his works and less than a third of his works have survived.

Although he was more famous as a medical practitioner, Galen was also a renowned philosopher of his times. He wrote extensively about logic and philosophy, and integrated philosophical thought with medical practice. His writings were influenced by earlier Greek and Roman thinkers, including Plato, Aristotle, and the Stoics.

5

Middle Ages (500–1400 AD)

Doctors in the Middle Ages knew little of the origination for the ailments that they were trying to treat, and not knowing the cause of the ailment made it incredibly difficult to try and figure out a way to treat or prevent it. Most doctors came from the higher end of the social ladder, and were generally more educated. Since the lower class consisted mostly of farmers or servants, their education level was extremely limited. The small amount of information that was available about the medical field made it impossible for doctors in the Middle Ages to properly practice medicine. There was almost no literature available and the literature that could be found was often written in a language that would need to be translated. The fact that the literature was being translated left a large margin of error. People did not travel or learn from other cultures the way that we do today, and that lack of knowledge led to the detriment of the medical field.

Many of the medical practices that existed during this period are no longer used today. Since there was little research done on the human body almost all physicians relied on the literature that was developed by Galen's observations of the human anatomy. This meant that there were many beliefs that were not accurate. Doctors in the Middle Ages had no way of knowing, if it was their practices of the disease itself that was hurting the patient!

Successful cures in that era were what today seem to be crazy cures. For example:

• Bleeding, applying leeches, smelling strong posies or causing purging or vomiting

- Cutting open buboes, draining the pus and making the patient hot or cold, e.g. by taking hot baths
- Trepanning—cutting a hole in the skull
- Praying, or whipping themselves to try to earn God's forgiveness
- Lighting fires in rooms and spreading the smoke, tidying rubbish from the streets and banning new visitors to towns and villages

Instruments used for managing a patient were often little more than kitchen utensils or something that could be created fairly easily!

Bloodletting was a tactic that was commonly used by doctors in the Middle Ages. It was a process in which doctors would make certain incisions and drain a certain amount of blood from the patient's body. The doctors believed that this was allowing the tainted blood to leave the body so that fresh clean blood could come and replace it. The biggest problems associated with it were that either the incision often became infected or too much blood would be drained from the patient resulting in death.

The practice of medicine in the Middle Ages was rooted in the Greek tradition. **Hippocrates**, the "Father of Medicine", described the body as made up of four humours—yellow bile, phlegm, black bile, and blood—and controlled by the four elements—fire, water, earth, and air. Many diseases were thought to be caused by an excess of blood in the body and bloodletting was seen as the obvious cure. Another important aspect in the treatment of ailments was diet. The food choices have an important impact on health—this was known since antiquity. "Let food be thy medicine and medicine be thy food" is a quote from Hippocrates found in his medical writings.

Later the Greek concept of the four humours was revised by **Galen**. It evolved into a theory of temperament, which accounted for psychological and social as well as physical characteristics.

It was a period of mixture of existing ideas from antiquity and spiritual influences.

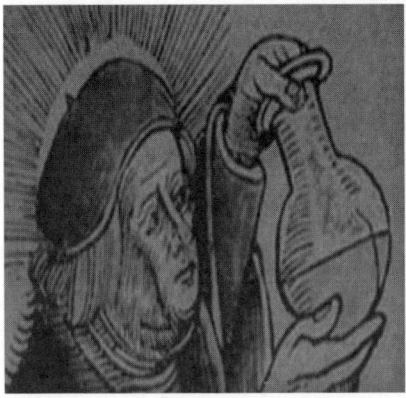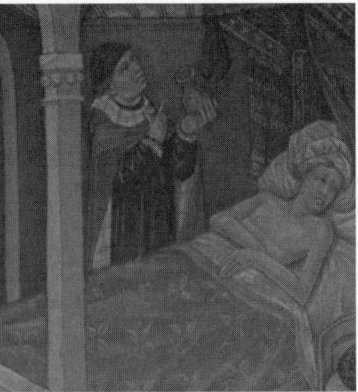

Fig. 10: Urine inspection was the most common method of diagnosis in Middle Ages. So much so that the urine flask became the symbol of the doctor just like stethoscope in present times

On one end observation, palpation, feeling the pulse, and urine examination would be the tools of the doctor. Urine inspection was the most common method of diagnosis and the urine flask became the symbol of the doctor (Fig. 10). [In present time, of course, the stethoscope is the symbol of the doctor, but that too may change in future! In order to better observe their patients' urine, doctors invented round-bottomed glass flasks. Interestingly, according to one English physician, the urine of a diabetic tastes "wonderfully sweet as if it were imbued with honey or sugar."

Surgery such as amputations, cauterization,removal of cataracts, dental extractions, and even trepanning were practiced. Surgeons relied on opiates for anaesthesia and doused wounds with wine as a form of antiseptic. Many people sought out the local healer for care, or went to barber to be bled or even leeched! Midwives took care of childbirth and childhood ailments.

On the other end, the **Roman Catholic Church** effectively dominated the medical world. Any view different from the established Roman Catholic view was labelled heresy and punished accordingly. The Roman Catholic Church stated that illnesses were punishments from God and those who were ill were so because they were sinners. Suffering was seen as part of the human condition. As people became obsessed with their souls, they neglected their bodies. Medicine became a matter of faith and prescriptions became prayers. Medicine became steeped in superstition. Ideas about the origin and cure of disease were based on factors such as destiny, sin, and heavenly influences.

It was believed that the moon had the greatest influence on fluids on earth, and that it was the moon that had the ability to affect positively or negatively the four elements in the body. A knowledge of location of the moon and planets was considered important while making a diagnosis and deciding on a course of treatment. Physicians needed to know when to treat a patient and when not to, and the position of the planets determined this. A so-called **Zodiac Chart** also determined when bloodletting should be done as it was believed by some that the moon and planets determined this as well. Medical charts informed physicians what not to do for people born under a certain astrology sign.

Some of the most notorious illnesses of the Middle Ages were the **plague (the Black Death), leprosy,** and **Saint Anthony's fire.** Rich and poor succumbed to them with terrifying speed. **Leprosy** was very disfiguring and, therefore, sufferers were feared and kept apart. Lepers were obliged to live outside a town or village and to carry a bell to warn people of their approach.

Plague (the Black Death) was one of the most devastating pandemics in human history. The sufferers were covered in mysterious black boils that oozed blood and pus and gave the illness its name, the "Black Death." It is thought to have started in China or central Asia before spreading west. It swept through the Mediterranean region and Europe in the 13th and 14th centuries. It took over 150 years for Europe's population to recover. The plague reoccurred occasionally in Europe until the 19th century. The aftermath of the plague created a series of religious, social, and economic upheavals which had profound effects on the course of European history.

In **St. Anthony's fire** the sufferers were afflicted with burning extremities. It was caused by the ingestion of tainted rye. As it progressed, the bright red extremities—hands, feet and whole limbs—could become gangrenous and fall off. There were many Antonine hospitals to which patients flocked. These hospitals, dedicated to Saint Anthony Abbot, gave patients a mixture called Saint Vinage and cooling herbs such as verbena and sage were applied to soothe the burning heat. Amputations of the affected limbs were also performed.

Herbs, flowers, and perfumes formed a large part of everyday life and were inextricably linked with magic and medicine. Medicinal plants and herbs were an important and major part in the pharmacopeia. Medicines were made from herbs, spices, and resins. Dioscorides, a Greek, wrote his Materia Medica in 65 AD.

Headache and aching joints were treated with sweet-smelling herbs such as rose, lavender, sage, and hay. A mixture of henbane and hemlock was applied to aching joints. Coriander was used to reduce fever. Stomach pains and sickness were treated with wormwood, mint, and balm. Lung problems were treated with a medicine made of liquorice and comfrey. Cough syrups and drinks were prescribed for chest and head-colds and coughs. Wounds were cleaned and vinegar was widely used as a cleansing agent as it was believed that it would kill disease. Mint was used in treating venom and wounds. Myrrh was used as an antiseptic on wounds.

There was no experimentation to test the efficacy of a particular herb treatment on ailments. If successful, it was ascribed to their action upon the humors within the body and the belief that such natural herbal remedies must have been intended for such purpose by God. In fact there was no tradition of scientific medicine, and observations went hand in hand with spiritual and religious influences.

The Middle Age was in fact the period of 'Dark Age' in the history of medicine.

Period of Renaissance (1400–1700 AD)

Renaissance medicine is the term used for the development of medicine at the time of the Renaissance in Europe. The renaissance period started in northern Italy during the 14th century and spread to Europe in the late 15th century. It starts from the date of discovery of America by Columbus. The renaissance period of new thinking changed the culture of the English people. Poets and philosophers, painters and musicians, mathematicians and scientists appeared in numbers and swept off age long superstitions and dogmas from the minds of the people and pointed to an age of reasoning and rational approach to the problems of humanity. Although very few people could read and write, ideas flourished and the newly invented printing press was a revolution in information technology which resulted in spread of ideas and knowledge around Europe as never before.

The main change in Renaissance medicine was largely due to the increase in anatomical knowledge, aided by an easing of the legal and cultural restrictions on dissecting cadavers. This allowed doctors to gain a much better understanding of the human body and get rid of techniques that harmed rather than cured. Previously, the church had banned dissection, believing that it was against dignity of the deceased, who should be buried whole.

There was transmission of knowledge from the middle east, where muslim scholars had made some major advances in the treatment of disease and injury. Some of this knowledge filtered into Europe when scholars fled muslim lands as the Islamic dominion collapsed, but much was brought back from the Crusades (the Crusades were a series of military campaigns against the muslims of the middle east). Here, the advanced techniques used by Islamic doctors to treat injuries and lessen the impact of disease impressed the crusaders, many of whom brought this knowledge back when they returned to Europe.

The church still dominated medicine, understanding the organs and systems of the human body. The church did not permit the dissection of 'God fearing bodies' so it was often the bodies of criminals or 'sinners' that were used. Physicians continued to refine their knowledge of anatomy and scrutinized how the human body works from watching these dissections. Sometimes the criminal was alive at the start of proceedings as part of their punishment! During the Renaissance, the human body was regarded as a creation of God and the ancient Greek view of the four humors prevailed. Accordingly it was still considered that sickness was due to an imbalance in these humors and treatments, such as bleeding the patient or inducing vomiting, were aimed at restoring the balance of these four humors.

The surgeons of this era were also categorized as a class system. They were acknowledged as master surgeons, "surgeons of the long robe," or the lower class of barber surgeons, "surgeons of the short robe"!

Discoveries during the Renaissance laid the foundations for a change in thinking leading to the view that the body is made up of specialized systems that work together—the basis of medical knowledge that we still see today. As the understanding of the body increased, so did the development of new medicines. Building on knowledge of herbs and minerals, renaissance pharmacists experimented with new plants brought from distant lands by explorers like **Christopher Columbus**. The bark of the Quina tree contained an ingredient called quinine which is still used in the treatment of malaria. The leaves of the tobacco plant were thought to have medicinal properties, although we now know it is responsible for an enormous number of deaths. Laudanum, an opium-based painkiller, was prescribed for many disorders and remained in use until Victorian times.

IMPORTANT PERSONALITIES IN THE FIELD OF MEDICINE DURING RENAISSANCE PERIOD

LEONARDO DA VINCI

He was originally a god gifted artist.

His research centered around his desire to learn more about how the human brain processes visual and sensory information and how that connects to the soul.

He was first to demonstrate the ventricles of brain by wax injection and to depict correctly the foetus and its membrane within the uterus. Originally, he studied the bones and muscles in relation to art. He pursued his investigation to study the deeper parts of the body, viscera, brain blood vessels and more specially the heart.

He believed that visual information entered the body through the eye and then continued by sending nerve impulses through the optic nerve, and eventually reaching the soul.

Leonardo da Vinci believed the ancient notion that the soul was housed in the brain.

He did research on the role of the spinal cord in humans by studying frogs. He noted that as soon as the frog's medulla of the spine is broken, the frog would die. This led him to believe that the spine is the basis for the sense of touch, cause of movement, and the origin of nerves. As a result of his studies on the spinal cord, he also came to the conclusion that all peripheral nerves begin from the spinal cord.

Da Vinci also did some research on the sense of smell. He is credited with being the first to define the olfactory nerve as one of the cranial nerves.

Leonardo da Vinci made his anatomical sketches based on observing and dissecting 30 cadaveres. His sketches were very detailed and included organs, muscles of superior extremity, the hand, and the skull.

Leonardo was well known for his three-dimensional drawings (Fig. 11). His anatomical drawings were not found until 380 years after his death! Though his artwork was

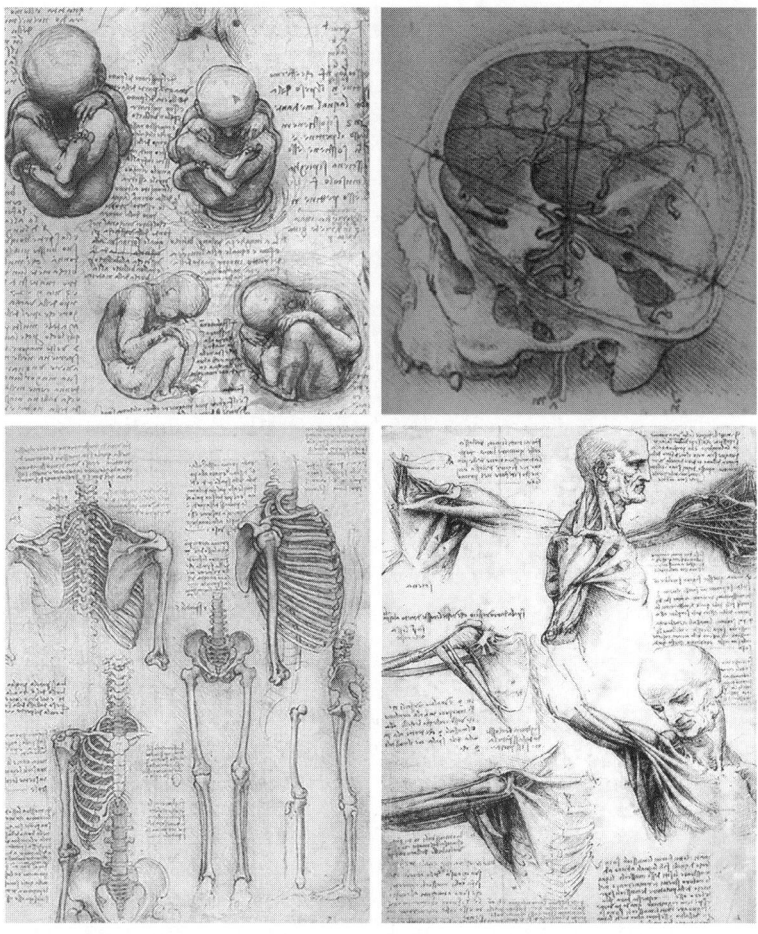

Fig. 11: 3D anatomical drawings by Leonardo da Vinci

widely observed before, some of his original research was not made public until the 20th century.

PARACELSUS

Paracelsus was the most disputed person of the time in the 16th century. His father was a physician and he practiced in a number of mining towns. As a boy he learned some practical medicine at home through observing his father. It is likely that he learned some folk medicine as well. He also picked up some alchemy (magical and secretive use of

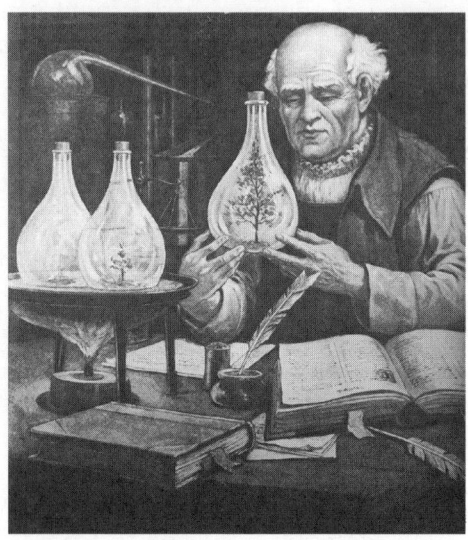

philosopher's stone, which was supposed to possess many valuable attributes such as the power to heal, to prolong life, and to change lead into gold; philosopher's stone was not a literal stone but instead a wax, liquid, or powder that held magical powers) from his father who had an interest in the subject. As a boy in mining towns, he would have observed metallurgical practices as well as the diseases that afflicted the men who worked the mines.

Traditionally, it has been said that Paracelsus was taught by several bishops. At the age of fourteen he left home to begin a long period of wandering. He apparently visited a number of universities, but there is no proof that he ever took a medical degree. As an adult, however, he picked up practical medical knowledge by working as a surgeon in a number of the mercenary armies that ravaged Europe in the seemingly endless wars of the period. He wrote that he visited most of the countries of Central, Northern, and Eastern Europe.

It is only in the final fifteen years of his life that the records of his travels become clearer. In 1527, he was called to Basel to treat a leg ailment of the famed publisher of humanist classics, Johannes Frobenius. In Basel Paracelsus also gave medical advice to the Dutch scholar Erasmus and came in contact with some of the more prominent scholars of the religious reformation. He was appointed city physician and professor of medicine. But although he was permitted to lecture at the University of Basel, he had no official appointment with the medical faculty there. He was a voluminious writer and himself predicted that his writing may be understood 20 years after his death.

Paracelsus became a figure of dispute and hatred for scorning conservative physicians of the university. On the occasion of the St. John's Day bonfire, he threw Avicenna's revered Canon of medicine to the blaze! There was so much hatred for him that when one of his patient died, a disastrous lawsuit followed and he left Basel in haste, even leaving behind his manuscripts.

Till final years of his life Paracelsus moved from town to town, and he often left his manuscripts behind as he had in Basel. He was an angry man who antagonized many of those he met—even those who tried to help him. In the end he was called to Salzburg to treat the bishop. There he died at the early age of forty-eight.

Paracelsus had chemical view of life. In his work he has mentioned 'paramirum sulphur, mercury, salt' meaning sulphur burns, mercury becomes smoke and salt becomes ash. According to his principle all diseases depend upon the maladjustment of the three.

AMBROISE PARÉ

He was a French surgeon, anatomist and an inventor of surgical instruments. He was a military surgeon during the French campaigns in Italy, in period 1533–36. It was here that, having run out of boiling oil (which was the accepted way of treating firearm wounds), Paré turned to an ancient Roman remedy: Turpentine, egg yolk and oil of roses. He applied it to the wounds and found that it relieved pain and sealed the wound effectively. He reformed surgical practice when he started using ligatures to stop bleeding, rather than painful procedure of cauterization. For the ligatures of arteries, he used silk threads to tie up the arteries of

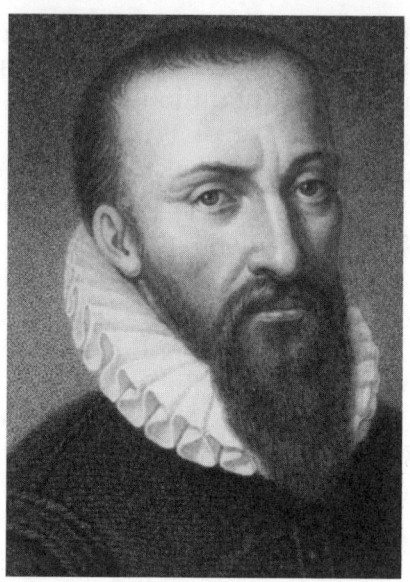

amputated limbs to try to stop the bleeding. As antiseptics had not yet been invented this method led to an increased fatality rate and was abandoned by medical professionals of that time. Additionally, Paré set up a school for midwives in Paris, and designed artificial limbs.

ANDREAS VESALIUS

He had a background of medical family. He was a professor of anatomy at Padua, Italy, in 1537. He had secretly collected

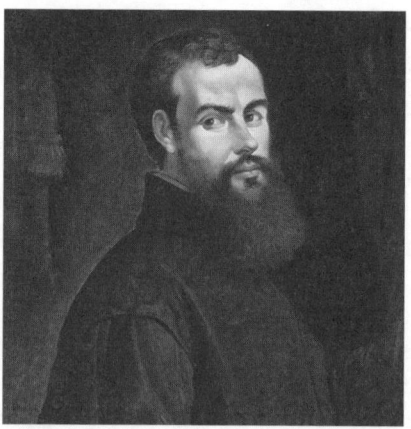

a skeleton of a criminal from a gallows (crossbar avoid for hanging criminals) outside the city wall! His dissections of the human body helped to rectify the misconceptions made in ancient times, particularly by Galen, who (for religious reasons) had been able only to study animals such as dogs and monkeys. He wrote many books on anatomy from his observations; his best-known work was De Humani Corporis Fabrica, published in 1543, which contained detailed drawings of the human body posed as if alive. Through his figures he represented body in action. He portrayed that the lower jaw consisted of a single bone and the sternum was composed only of three parts. He observed valves of vein and that each artery supplying a viscus is accompained by a vein. In the first edition of his book he depicted the existance of minute pores in the interventricular septum, but in 1555, he changed his viewpoint by depicting no pores. Vasalius was succeeded by Realdus Columbus (1510–1599) who succeeded in demonstrating pulmonary circulation. It was published in his book Dere Anatomica in 1557.

Vasalius changed how human anatomy was viewed and researched. He is considered a legacy in the medical world. Nicolaus Copernicus published his book on planetary motion in 1543, one month before Vesalius published his work on anatomy (Fig. 12). The work by Copernicus overturned the medieval belief that the earth lay at the center of the universe, and the work by Vesalius overturned the old authorities about the structure of the human body. In 1543, these two separate books fostered a change in understanding of the place of mankind within the macrocosmic structure of the universe and the microcosmic structure of the human body.

WILLIAM HARVEY

He was an English medical doctor–physicist, known for his contributions in heart and blood movement. In 1626, he made a huge breakthrough by studying dying dogs, showing that the heart pumped blood around the body and that the heart had two distinct beating halves. This discovery that blood circulated around the body (Fig. 13) changed medical

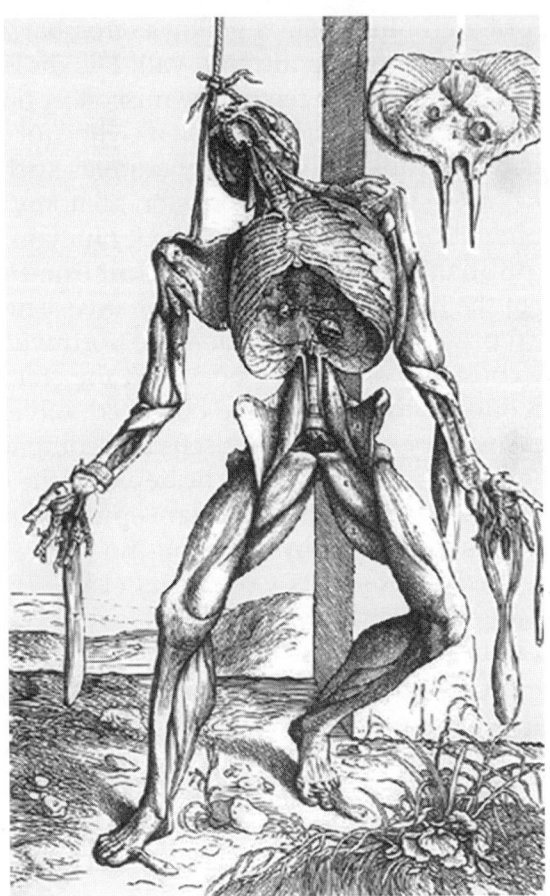

Fig. 12: Anatomical studies of Vasalius on skeleton of criminals hanged

practice and finally sounded the death knell for the harmful practice of bloodletting by barber surgeons. It also showed that the body contained specialized systems with different functions, all of which worked together in coordination to maintain life, a discovery that led to belief that the body was little more than a machine.

'The Motu Cordis' contains his extensive work on the body's circulation. This work opens up with clear definitions of Anatomy as well as types of Anatomy which clearly outlined a universal meaning of these words for other Renaissance physicians. Anatomy, as defined by him meant

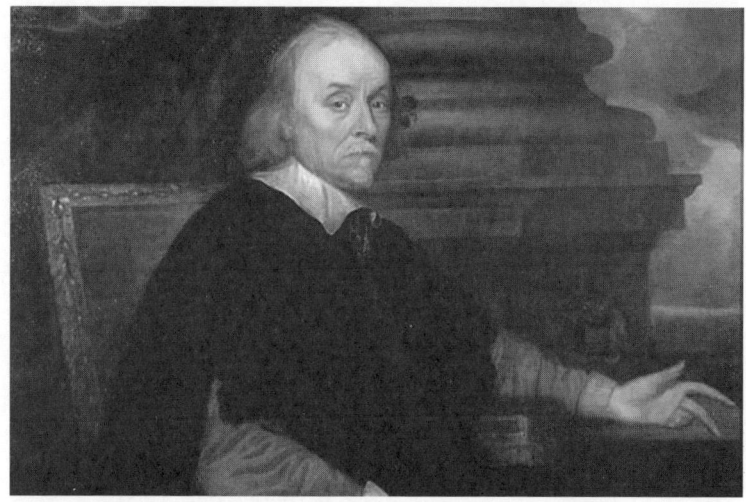

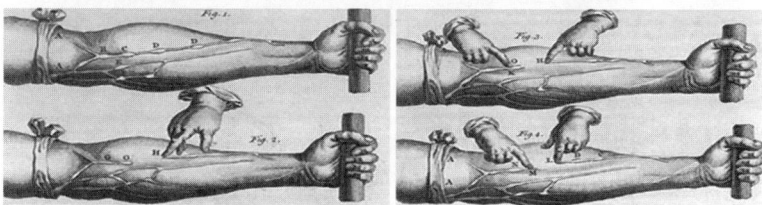

Fig. 13: Blood circulation depicted by William Harvey

'to be able to identify the actions or roles each part of the body plays in the overall function of the body by dissection, followed by visual identification.'

HIERONYMUS FABRICIUS

He was an anatomist and surgeon who prepared a human and animal anatomy atlas 'Tabulae Pictae' (Fig. 14). This work includes illustrations from many different artists and Fabricius is credited for providing a turning point in anatomical illustration. Fabricius' illustrations were of natural size and natural colours. After Fabricius' death, 'Tabulae pictae' disappeared and was not again discovered until 1909. Fabricius focused on the human brain and the fissures that are inside brain. In 'Tabulae pictae', he described the cerebral fissure that separates the temporal lobe from

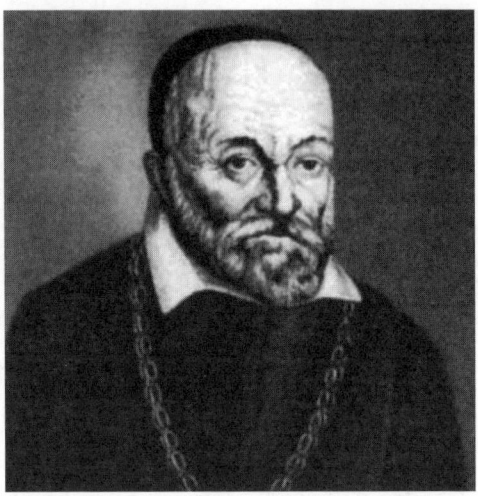

the frontal lobe. He also studied veins and was the first to discover the valves inside of veins.

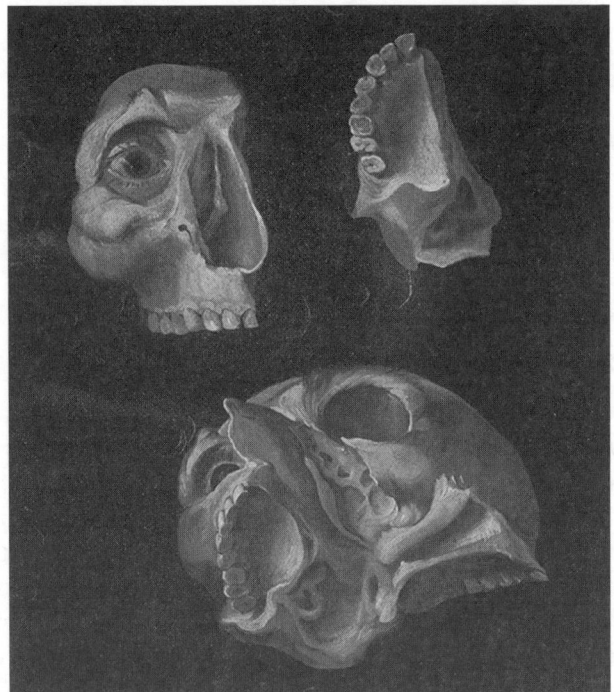

Fig. 14: From Tabulae pictae

PIERRE FRANCO

He was first person to perform a subpubic lithotomy. He wrote an article on hernia. He achieved great success in operating cataract.

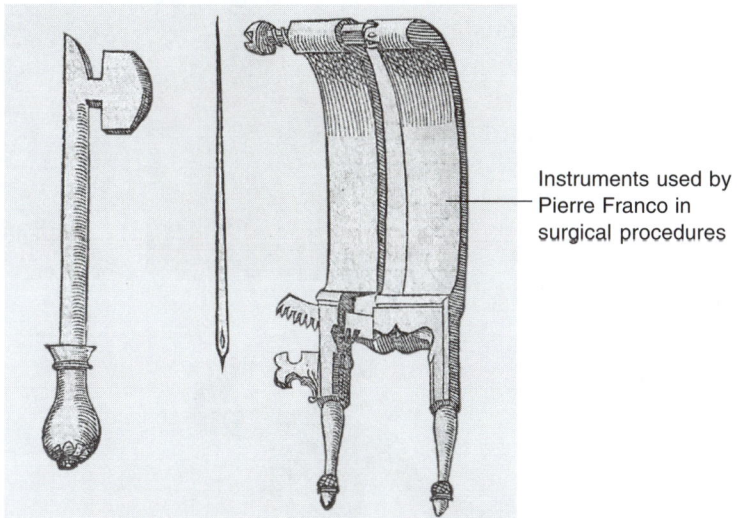

Instruments used by Pierre Franco in surgical procedures

GABRIEL FALLOPIUS

He is credited for his discovery of aqueduct and fallopian tubes during the period 1526–62.

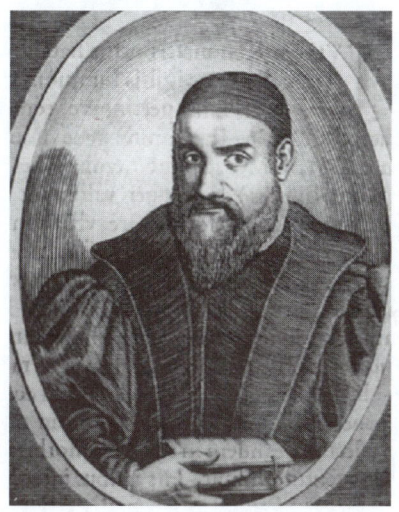

BARTOLOMEUS EUSTACHIUS

He was head of the Department of Anatomy at Rome. He was the first one to accurately illustrat eustachian tube, thoracic duct, cillary muscles, details of fascial muscles, larnyx and kidney (Fig. 15).

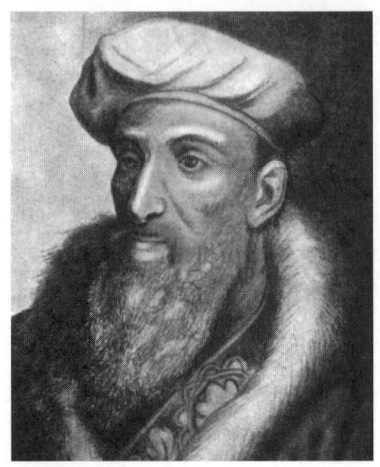

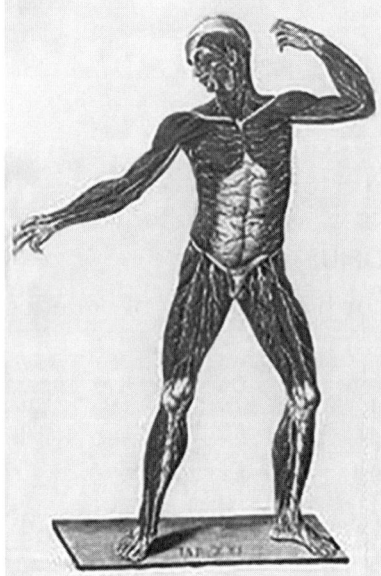

Fig. 15: Depiction of anatomy of human body by Eustachius

Women in Medicine

Catholic women played large roles in health and healing in medieval and early modern Europe. Rich families gave funds to convents and monasteries, and enrolled their daughters as nuns who provided free health services to the poor. Nursing was a religious role for women.

Modern Medicine (18th Century onwards)

In early modern times people started caring about dirt and disease. It was perceived that bad smells caused disease, this led them to do things which improved health, for example, cesspits were cleared regularly and housewives spent a lot of time boiling underclothes to keep them smelling nice. Interestingly, Queen Elizabeth I, bathed four times a day, whether she needed it or not! Her father, Henry VIII insisted that everyone at court was healthy, and courtiers were sent away even if they had a cold.

There was lot of focus on making the room and the patient smell nice. Doctors wore full bodysuits, with a 'beak' that was crammed with herbs, so that they would not smell a bad smell! New drugs like quinine, were discovered but doctors did not know how or why they worked. Tobacco was said to cure everything from wind to snake bites.

Superstitions such as king's touch would cure the disease of scrofula (a disease with glandular swellings, probably a form of tuberculosis), also known as 'King's evil' , prevailed.

18th century was harbinger of the 'Age of Enlightenment'. The practice of medicine changed in the face of rapid advances in science, as well as new approaches by physicians. In hospitals, doctors began much more systematic analysis of patients' symptoms for diagnosis. Among the more powerful new techniques were anaesthesia, and the development of both antiseptic and aseptic operating theatres. Effective cures were developed for certain endemic infectious diseases. However, the decline in many of the lethal diseases was due more to improvements in public health and nutrition than advances in medicine.

Medicine was revolutionized in the 19th century and beyond by advances in chemistry, laboratory techniques, and equipment. Old ideas of infectious disease epidemiology were gradually replaced by advances in bacteriology and virology.

In 1798, **Edward Jenner's** work on vaccinations, in particular for smallpox was a landmark in the development of preventative medicine (Fig. 16). He heard that milkmaids did not get smallpox but they did catch the much milder cowpox. Using careful scientific methods Jenner investigated and discovered that people who had cowpox did not get smallpox. Testing his theory on a boy called James Phipps, he injected him with pus from the sores of Sarah Nelmes, a milkmaid with cowpox. Jenner then injected him with smallpox. James did not catch the disease. Parliament rewarded Jenner in 1802 and 1807. Vaccination was made free for infants in 1840 and compulsory in 1853.

In 1864, **Louis Pasteur** proved that germs caused disease. He proved there are germs in the air by sterilising water

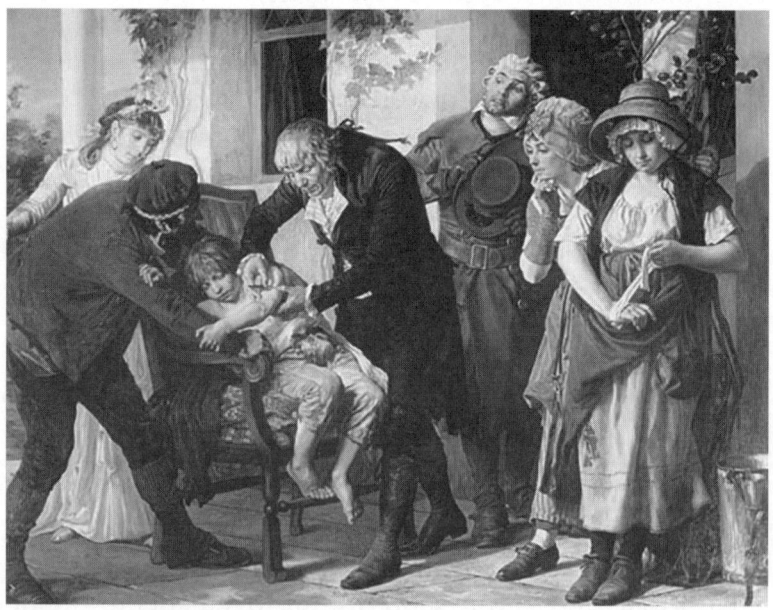

Fig. 16: Edward Jenner testing smallpox vaccine

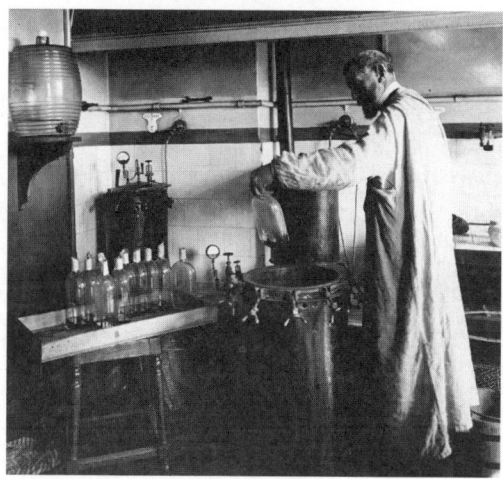

Fig. 17: Louis Pasteur working in his laboratory on 'germs'

and keeping it in a flask that did not allow airborne particles to enter (Fig. 17). This stayed sterile, but sterilised water kept in an open flask bred microbes again.

In 1884, **Robert Koch** discovered that bacteria caused diseases.

In 1880, **Charles Chamberland** discovered that injecting weakened germs inoculated the patient against that disease.

By 1900, scientists had discovered that viruses also caused diseases and malaria was carried by mosquitoes.

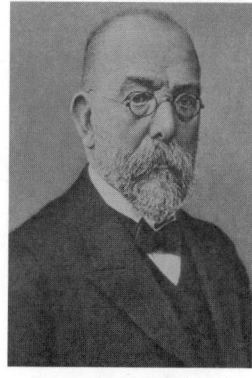
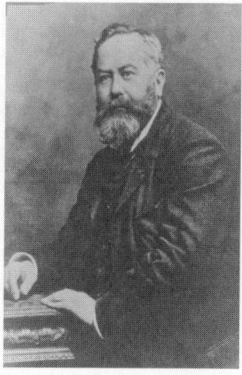
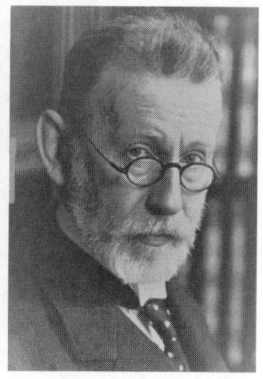

Robert Koch   Charles Chamberland   Paul Ehrlich

Researchers developed inoculations against rabies (1885), tuberculosis (1906) and diphtheria (1913).

In 1909, the German scientist **Paul Ehrlich** discovered that the chemical Salvarsan 606 cured syphilis.

At this point of history, it was for the first time that a patient had the prospect of going into hospital, undergoing an operation without pain or infection, and surviving!

The development of anaesthetics such as chloroform, discovered by **James Simpson** in 1847, greatly improved the success rate of surgery (Fig. 18). Though initially anaesthetics were not popular as they were uncomfortable for patients. Moreover, some doctors believed that pain was good for healing. Also at that time people did not understand how they worked and the side effects on the body were not properly recognised. The final breakthrough came when Queen Victoria accepted the use of chloroform as an anaesthetic during the delivery of her eighth child.

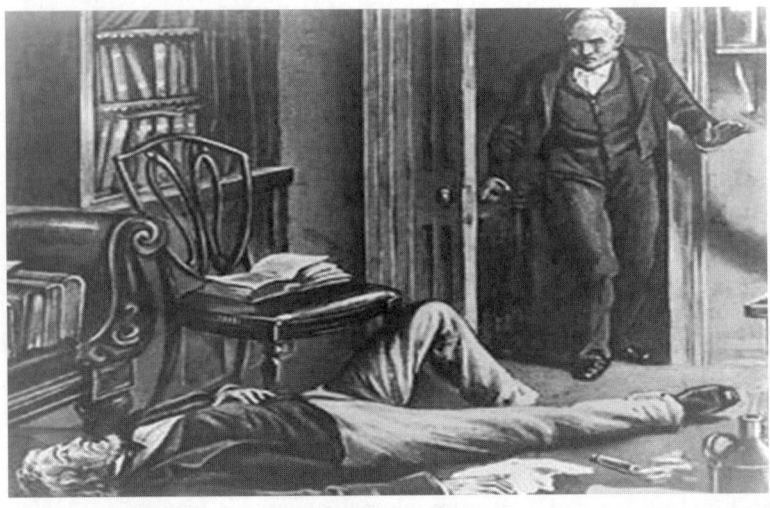

Fig. 18: James Simpson experimenting with chloroform for anaesthesia

Until Louis Pasteur's pioneering work on germ theory in the 1860s, surgeons left wounds unprotected. They reused bandages and rarely washed their hands or surgical equipment before operations. In 1864, **Joseph Lister** (Listerine mouthwash named after him) introduced an

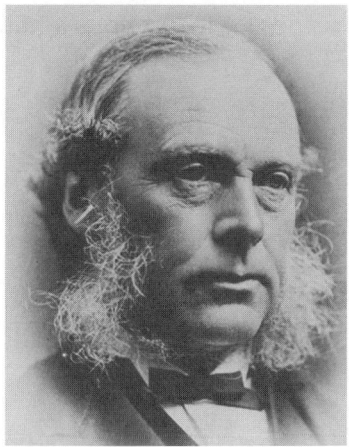

Joseph Lister—Listerine mouthwash named after him

antiseptic spray containing carbolic acid, that by 1866, reduced the death rate in patients by 45.7%. His spray was not used for long though, because carbolic acid actually damages the tissues and breathing it in causes many problems for doctor as well as patient. More successful was the special dressings he developed which contained carbolic acid to keep the wound clean. By the late 1890s Lister's antiseptic methods led to aseptic surgery and the introduction of sterile instruments in operating theatres. By 1898, rubber gloves were used and surgeon's hands were scrubbed clean beforehand.

After 1860, as a result of the work of **Florence Nightingale** there was upliftment in standards of nursing in Britain and also improvements in cleanliness in hospitals (Fig. 19). Majority of her time was spent working at old Barrack Hospital at Scutari, a district in Turkey. During her time the death rate there fell from 43 to 2%. This was solely attributed to her belief in prioritizing cleanliness and fresh air. Apart from this, it was her dedication that led to increased respect and reputation of nurses. She also worked for establishment of nursing training schools. By 1900, there were 64,000 trained nurses.

By the end of 19th century, surgeons were regularly doing successful internal operations, for example, appendectomies.

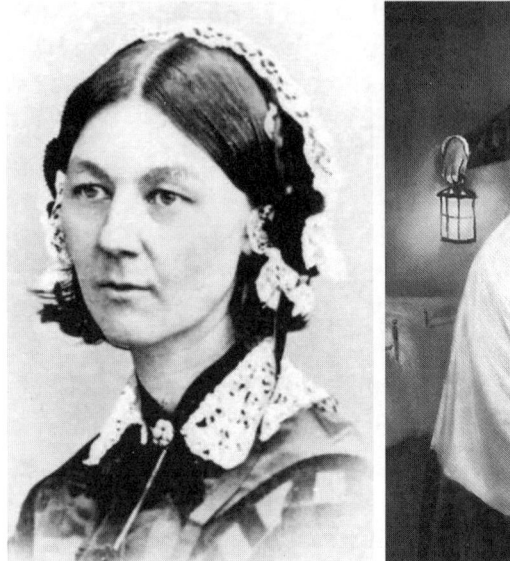
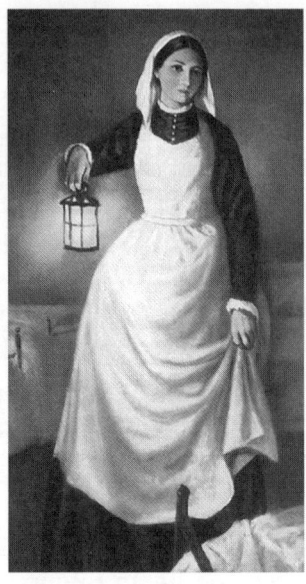

Fig. 19: Florence Nightangle—'Lady with the lamp'

X-rays (which were discovered in 1895) allowed doctors to see inside the body helping in the diagnosis and treatment of patients. Later **ultrasonic imaging, CT scanning, MR scanning** and other imaging methods became available.

In 1854, **John Snow** discovered the connection between contaminated water and cholera by plotting the course of a

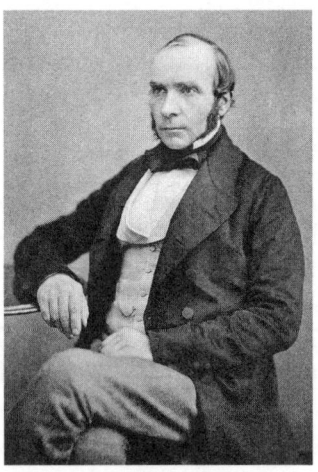

John Snow

cholera outbreak in the Broad Street area of London. He noticed that all the victims used the same water pump. When he removed the handle from the pump, the epidemic ended.

There is no time when it is 'good' to become ill, but the 20th century was a much better time to be ill than any previous period in history. By 1991, the average life expectancy of a man in Britain was 73, and that of a woman, 78!

Based on following spectacular scientific discoveries, doctors now understand the human body like never before.

- **Willem Einthoven** in Holland invented the electrocardiograph, or heart monitor in the early 1900s.
- **Karl Landsteiner** in Austria discovered blood groups in 1901.
- The discovery of **penicillin by Alexander Fleming**. Inspired by his work, **Florey and Chain** in the 1930s learned how to mass-produce penicillin—the first antibiotic (Fig. 20).
- The electron microscope was developed in 1931.
- **Francis Crick and James Watson** in Britain discovered the molecular structure of DNA in 1953 (Fig. 21).
- **Leroy Stevens** in America discovered **stem cells** in 1953.

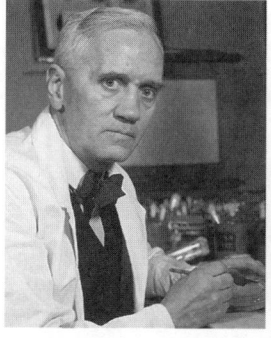
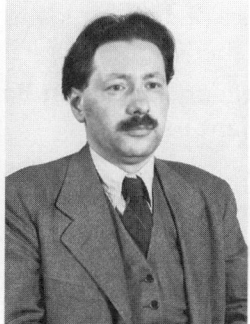
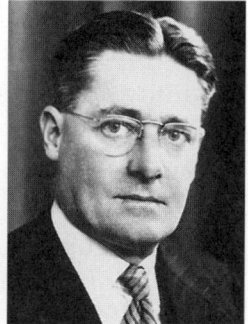

Alexander Fleming   Ernst Chain   Howard Florey

Fig. 20: All three were awarded Nobel Prize for discovery and manufacture of Penicillin in 1945

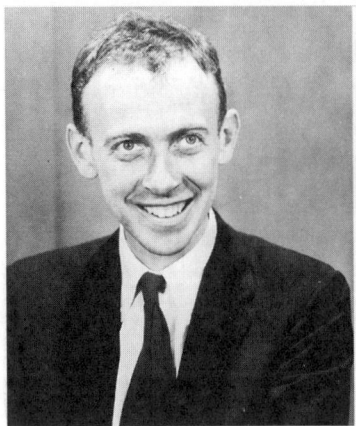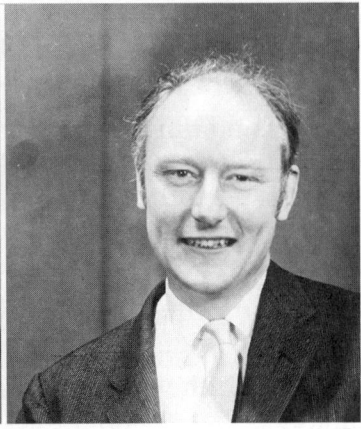

Fig. 21: Watson and Crick—discoverers of the molecular structure of DNA

- **Godfrey Hounsfield** in Britain invented the CAT scanner (a powerful X-ray machine that provides a cross-section of the human body) in 1972.
- **The Human Genome project** mapped all the 40,000 genes in the human body in the 1990s.
- The discovery of vitamins allowed doctors to cure diseases such as rickets.
- In 1922, the first clinical trials of injected insulin saved people with diabetes.
- British surgeon, **Archibald McIndoe,** did the **first plastic surgery** on the faces of disfigured airmen in the 1940s. They were nicknamed the 'Guinea Pig Club'.
- South African surgeon, **Christian Barnard,** performed the first heart transplant in 1967.
- **Louise Brown** became the first **'test-tube' baby** in 1978 (Fig. 22).
- **Laparoscopic surgery** or **'keyhole' surgery** technique, which avoided using large surgical cuts, became popular in the 1990s.
- **Remote surgery** is another recent development, with the Lindbergh operation in 2001 as a groundbreaking example.

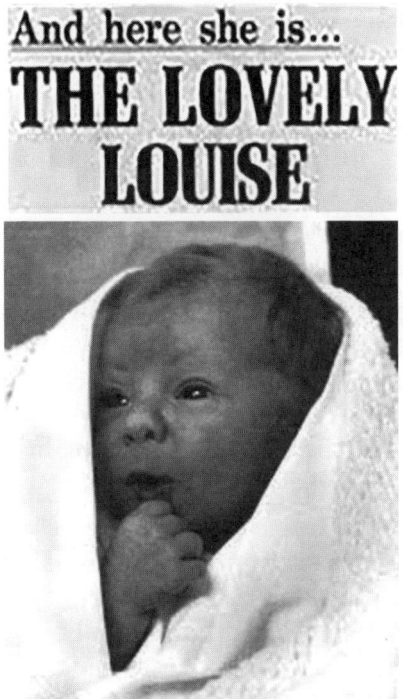

And here she is...
THE LOVELY LOUISE

Fig. 22: First test-tube baby—Louise Brown arrived in 1978

- **Oral rehydration therapy** has been extensively used since the 1970s to treat cholera and other diarrhea-inducing infections.

- The sexual revolution included taboo-breaking research in human sexuality such as the invention of hormonal contraception and the normalization of abortion and homosexuality in many countries. Family planning has promoted a demographic transition in most of the world. With threatening sexually transmitted infections use of barrier contraception has become imperative.

- Genetics have advanced with the discovery of the DNA molecule, **genetic mapping** and **gene therapy.** Stem cell research took off in the 2000s, **with stem cell therapy** as a promising method.

- **Evidence-based medicine** is a modern concept, not introduced to literature until the 1990s.

- **Prosthetics** have improved. In 1958, Arne Larsson in Sweden became the first patient to depend on an artificial cardiac pacemaker. He died in 2001 at age 86. Lightweight materials as well as neural prosthetics emerged in the end of the 20th century.

- Open-heart surgery was introduced for the first time in 1925. Cardiac surgery was further revolutionized 1948 onwards.

- In **1954 Joseph Murray, J. Hartwell Harrison** and others accomplished the first kidney transplantation. Transplantations of other organs, such as heart, liver and pancreas, were also introduced during the late 20th century. The first partial face transplant was performed in 2005, and the first full one in 2010.

- By the end of the 20th century, microtechnology had been used to create tiny robotic devices to assist microsurgery using micro-video and fiberoptic cameras to view internal tissues during surgery with minimally invasive practices.

INTERESTING NOTE ON ROLE OF NAZIS IN MODERN MEDICINE

The following experiments were done during the holocaust (World War II genocide of the European Jews, Fig. 23):

- **Freezing:** The experimental human subjects were dressed in pilot uniforms and dropped in freezing water that

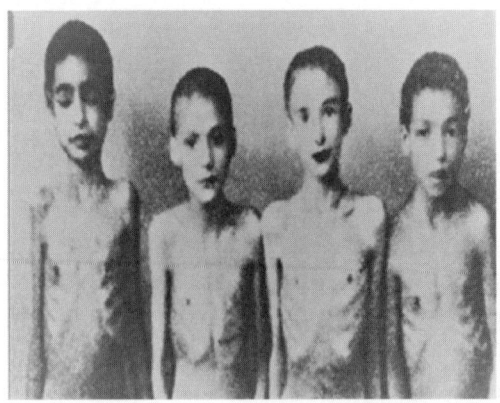

Fig. 23: Children victimized in Nazi experiments

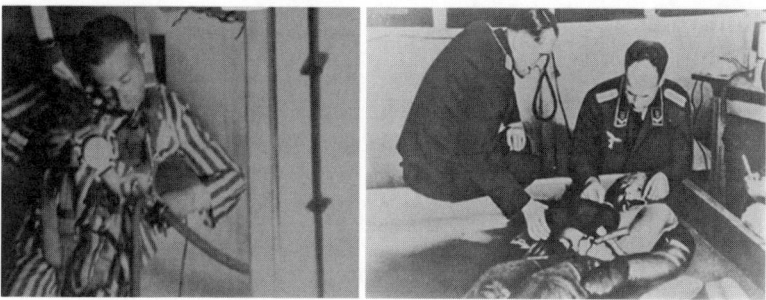

Fig. 24: Horrendous high altitude and freezing experiments

simulated conditions in the North Sea. Subjects' temperatures were taken rectally and rate of cooling was carefully charted (Fig. 24). Various methods for reheating hypothermic subject were employed and was theorized that sexual intercourse worked better than warm colonic irrigation!

- **Altitude and low-pressure effects:** The experimental human subjects were hung in parachutes and sealed inside a pressure chamber. To simulate low pressure air was pumped out of the chamber. It was observed that victims clawed at their faces and chewed their lips and tongues. Later their swollen brains were studied, some of them still living during the vivisection!

- **Deprivation of fresh water and dehyration:** Experimental human subjects were deprived of fresh water. Within days, they were observed to be licking the mopped floors for moisture! It was discovered that death from dehydration resembles high-speed kidney failure.

- **Sulfa antibiotics:** These antibiotics were tested by gashing the legs of experimental human subjects and rubbing in wood shavings, ground glass, and infected matter. To simulate gangrene, blood vessels were tied off or cut, and wounds were not allowed to heal. Later the body of experimental human subjects was autopsied to find how effective the drugs had been!

- Prisoners were splashed with **mustard gas** (which is actually an oily liquid) and various unscientific remedies were tested for effect on the chemical burns!

- **Burn treatments and grafting:** The experimental human subjects were exposed to burning phosphorous and then underwent burn treatments and grafting techniques without any anaesthesia!

- **Sterilization:** Experimental women were injected with mysterious compounds, now believed to be silver nitrate or iodine, which caused profuse vaginal bleeding and cervical cancer. Hysterectomies, vasectomies, castration and the removal of ovaries were attempted without any pain control method!

- **Twin studies:** During the study, a blue dye was injected into children's eyes and were stitched together to make sets of conjoined twins. Infectious agents were injected into one twin. When both subjects died because of infection, they were autopsied together!

What flashes in your mind about Hitler and Nazis? No doubt one would describe them as *brutal and inhumane*. They treated humans as laboratory rats. Virtually these experiments were nothing more than torturous death of human subjects. Moreover what little was discovered was either already known, or the research was done in such non-standard conditions that conclusions were not worth documentation.

But as a coin has two sides, the brighter side of this inhumane dictatorship in history is reflected by following:

- Nazi scientists correctly picked up on X-rays as a possible source of genetic damage.

- Hitler launched a huge campaign against tobacco and alcoholism (though Hitler's real gameplay behind it was to stop corruption of German germplasm by adoption of these vices which were propagated by Jews).

- Nazis identified the dangers of organochlorine pesticides such as DDT before other nations.

- Nazis established the link between asbestos and lung cancer.

- Nazis developed the first high-powered electron microscope.

- Nazi doctors promoted breast self-examination to detect tumors at an early stage.
- Hitler was a vegetarian and stressed on importance of vitamins, minerals, whole foods and fiber in diet of Nazis.
- The brutal experiments provide some of the most comprehensive data that's still occasionally cited. For example, no human subjects would ever volunteer to have their eardrums ruptured by low pressure! So the results of the experiments done during holocaust are still the gold standard for predicting high-altitude exposure results. Similarly in case of hypothermia experiments.
- Last but the most important contribution of Nazi medicine to modern medicine is that it has profoundly affected medical ethics. Today's ethical code of treating every person equally without regard to race or ethnic background and giving respect to human body are direct outgrowth of horrendous Nazi research work.

WOMEN AS PHYSICIANS AFTER THE ADVENT OF ERA OF MODERN MEDICINE

It was very difficult for women to become doctors in any field in early nineteenth century. It was a pity that women doctors, if any, were paid less than their male counterparts and sometimes even less than male factory workers!

ELIZABETH BLACKWELL AND ELIZABETH GARRETT ANDERSON

These two british women, born in 1821 and 1836 respectively, were instrumental not only in the emancipation of women but also for admitting of women to the medical profession.

In 1876, the Act of Parliament allowed women to enter the medical profession. Elizabeth Blackwell was the first to graduate as an MD in America and later **first to get enrolled onto UK Medical Register**. Elizabeth Garrett Anderson became the first woman to qualify as a doctor in Britain and **second to get enrolled onto UK Medical Register**. They opened schools of medicine, worked with Florence Nightingale, trained future generations of doctors and tirelessly supported women's rights all their lives.

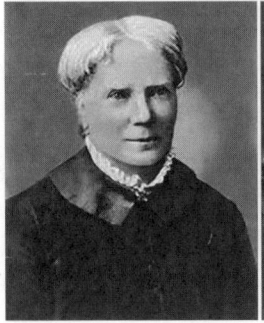 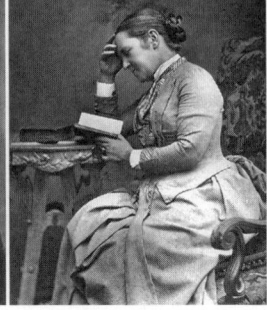 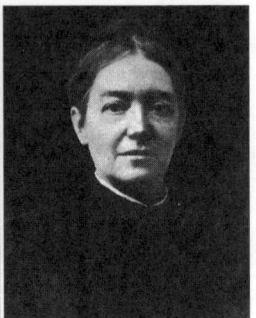

Elizabeth Blackwell   Elizabeth Garrett   Mary Putnam Jacobi
                             Anderson

They both felt a moral imperative, not only to fulfil their own ambitions and desires but to give back to society, to improve and help society as a whole to develop. Elizabeth Blackwell went as far as to say "If society will not admit of woman's free development, then society must be remodelled" and Elizabeth Garrett Anderson became England's first female mayor in 1908. Sadly, neither of the two lived to see full voting rights for women in the UK or the US.

While Blackwell viewed medicine as a means for social and moral reform, her student **Mary Putnam Jacobi** (1842–1906) focused on curing disease. At a deeper level of disagreement, Blackwell felt that women would succeed in medicine because of their humane female values, but Jacobi believed that women should participate as the equals of men in all medical specialties using identical methods, values and insights.

Even after Blackwell had broken the barrier to medical education, women students faced obstacles like that of exclusion from hospital training and practice.

Interestingly, in 1892, the University of Johns Hopkins was committed to establish a model medical school, but it did not have sufficient funds. A group of prominent women raised $100,000 and offered to the University with the condition of permitting admission to women in medical school on same basis as men. The trustees offered to open the school to women if the grant was increased to $500,000. The group succeeded in raising the money and then insisted on raising the admission standards to include a bachelors' degree, knowledge of French and German and premedical studies. The faculty and trustees although considered these criteria too demanding, agreed to them reluctantly. As a result, in 1896, 33% of the students at Johns Hopkin Medical School were women.

Later, due to educational reforms, stricter licensing and financial difficulties, many medical schools returned to policy of denying admission to women. In 1916, at John Hopkins Medical School, only 10% of the students were women.

By 1970s, the awareness of sex discrimination heightened followed by agitation for equal right to education for women. The result was that by 1990s, 40% of medical students in various schools and 18% of all practicing physicians were women.

Unforgettable Indian Names in the Field of Medicine

FROM HISTORY

BIDHAN CHANDRA ROY

Bidhan Chandra Roy **(1st July 1882–1st July 1962)** was an eminent Indian physician, educationist, philanthropist, freedom fighter and politician who served as the Chief Minister of West Bengal from 1948 until his death in 1962. He is often considered the Maker of Modern West Bengal due to his key role in the founding of several institutions and five eminent cities, Durgapur, Kalyani, Bidhannagar, Ashokenagar and Habra. He is one of the few people in history to has obtained FRCS and MRCP degrees simultaneously.

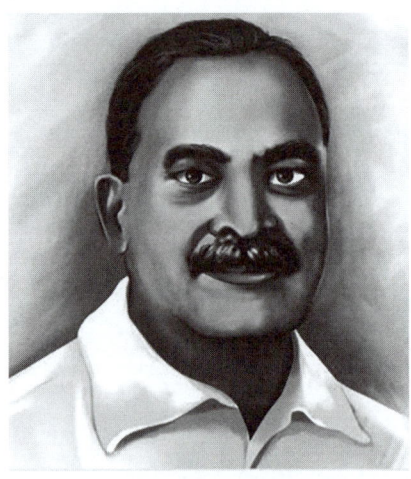

He was born to a Bengali Kayastha family on 1st July 1882 at Bankipore, Patna, Bihar, where his father, Prakash

Chandra Roy, was working as an excise inspector. His mother, Aghore Kamini Devi, was a pious lady and a devoted social worker. He was the youngest of five siblings—he had two sisters and two brothers. His parents were ardent Brahmo Samajists, led an austere and disciplined life, and devoted their time and money to the service of everyone in need, irrespective of caste or creed.

After completing his matriculation from Patna Collegiate School in 1897, he obtained his IA degree from Presidency College, Calcutta, and BA from Patna College with Honors in Mathematics. After completing his graduation in mathematics, he applied for admission to the Indian Institute of Engineering Science and Technology (IIEST) and the Calcutta Medical College. His application was accepted by both institutions and he opted to pursue medical studies. The partition of Bengal was announced while he was in college. Opposition to the partition was being organised by nationalist leaders like Lala Lajpat Rai, Bal Gangadhar Tilak and Bipin Chandra Pal. Bidhan resisted the immense pull of the movement. He controlled his emotions and concentrated on his studies, realising that he could serve his nation better by qualifying in his profession first.

Intending to enroll himself at St Bartholomew's Hospital to pursue postgraduate study in medicine, he set sail to England in February 1909 with only ₹1200. However, the Dean of St. Bartholomew's Hospital was reluctant to accept an Asian student and rejected Bidhan's application. He did not lose heart but kept submitting his application again and again till the Dean, after 30 admission requests, admitted him to the college. He completed his postgraduation in just two years and three months, and in May 1911, accomplished the rare feat of becoming a member of the Royal College of Physicians and a fellow of the Royal College of Surgeons simultaneously. After this he joined the Provincial Health Service. He exhibited immense dedication and hard work, and would even serve as a nurse when necessary. In his free time he practiced privately, charging a nominal fee.

Following his return from England after postgraduation in 1911, he taught at the Calcutta Medical College, and later at the Campbell Medical School and the Carmichael Medical College.

Dr Roy believed that 'swaraj' (the call to action for India's freedom) would remain a dream unless the people were healthy and strong in mind and body. He made contributions to the organisation of medical education. He played an important role in the establishment of the Jadavpur TB Hospital, Chittaranjan Seva Sadan, Kamala Nehru Memorial Hospital, Victoria Institution (college), and Chittaranjan Cancer Hospital. The Chittaranjan Seva Sadan for women and children was opened in 1926. Women were unwilling to come to the hospital initially, but due to Dr Roy and his team's hardwork, the Seva Sadan was embraced by women of all classes and communities. He opened a center for training women in nursing and social work.

In 1942, Rangoon fell to Japanese bombing and caused an exodus from Calcutta fearing Japanese insurgency. Dr Roy was serving as the Vice-Chancellor of the University of Calcutta. He acquired air-raid shelters for schools and college students to have their classes in, and provided relief for students, teachers and employees alike. In recognition for his efforts, the Doctorate of Science was conferred upon him in 1944.

He believed that the youth of India would determine the future of the nation. He felt that the youth must not take part in strikes and fasts but should study and commit themselves to social work.

The nation honoured him with the Bharat Ratna on 4th February 1961. On 1st July 1962, his 80th birthday, after treating his morning patients and discharging affairs of the state, he took a copy of the 'Brahmo Geet' and sang a piece from it. Few hours later he died at midday past three.

In India, the National Doctors' Day is celebrated in his memory every year on 1st July. The BC Roy National Award was instituted in 1962 in Dr Roy's memory and has been awarded annually since 1976. The award recognizes excellent contributions in the areas of medicine, politics, science, philosophy, literature and arts. The Dr BC Roy Memorial

Library and Reading Room for Children in the Children's Book Trust, New Delhi, was opened in 1967.

RAM NATH CHOPRA

Sir Ram Nath Chopra **(17th August 1882–13th June 1973)** is "Father of Indian Pharmacology".

He was born in Jammu and Kashmir region. After finishing his school and college in Lahore, he went to England in 1903 and qualified in the Natural Sciences Tripos. He stood third in the examination for the Indian Medical Service. In 1922, he was appointed Professor, Department of Pharmacology at the Calcutta School of Tropical Medicine.

He had keen interest in indigenous drugs and had a vision that India should have self-sufficient drug resources. He was the pioneer to conduct researches on herbal remedies including Rauwolfia serpentina. He headed the Drugs Enquiry Committee of 1930-31 which examined the need for imports, control and legislation.

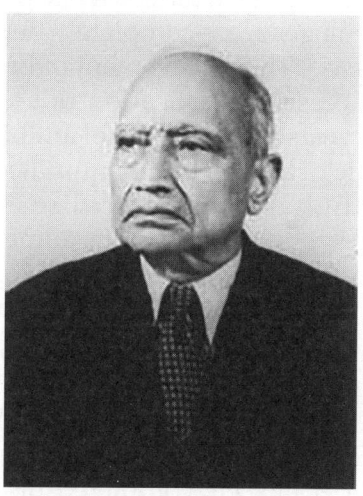

UPENDRANATH BRAHMACHARI

Rai Bahadur Sir Upendranath Brahmachari **(19th December 1873–6th February 1946)** was an Indian scientist and a leading medical practitioner of his time. He synthesised Urea Stibamine (carbostibamide) in 1922 and determined that it

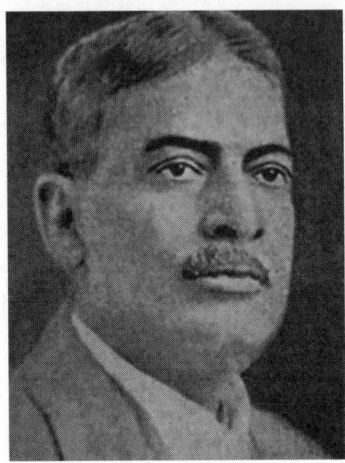

was an effective substitute for the other antimony-containing compounds in the treatment of kala-azar (visceral leishmaniasis) which is caused by a protozoon, *Leishmania donovani*. His discovery led to the saving of thousands of lives in India, particularly in the erstwhile province of Assam, where several villages were completely depopulated by the devastating disease. The achievement of Brahmachari was a milestone in successful application of science in medical treatment in the years before arrival of antibiotics, when there were few specific drugs, including quinine for malaria, iron for anaemia, digitalis for heart diseases and arsenic compounds for syphilis. Most other ailments were treated symptomatically by palliative methods. Urea Stibamine was thus a significant addition to the arsenal of specific medicines.

Upendranath Brahmachari was born on 19th December 1873 in Sardanga village near Purbasthali, District-Burdwan of West Bengal, India. His father, Nilmony Brahmachari,was a physician in East Indian Railways. His mother's name was Saurabh Sundari Devi. He completed his early education from Eastern Railways Boys' High School, Jamalpur. In 1893, he passed BA degree from Hooghly Mohsin College with honours in Mathematics and Chemistry. Thereafter, he went to study medicine with higher chemistry. He passed his master's degree in 1894 from the Presidency College, Kolkata. In MB Examination of 1900 of the University of Calcutta, he stood first in Medicine and in Surgery for which he received Goodeve and Macleod awards. He obtained his MD degree in 1902, and was awarded a PhD degree in 1904, for his research paper on "Studies in Haemolysis" both from the University of Calcutta.

Brahmachari joined the Provincial Medical Service in September 1899, and appointed as a teacher of Pathology and Materia Medica, and physician in the Dacca Medical School in 1901. In 1905, he was appointed as a teacher in Medicine and Physician at the Campbell Medical School (now Nilratan Sircar Medical College and Hospital), Calcutta, where he carried out most of his work on kala-azar and made his monumental discovery of Urea Stibamine. In 1923, he joined as Additional Physician in the Medical College Hospital. He retired from the government service as a physician in 1927. After retirement from the government service Brahmachari joined the Carmichael Medical College in Kolkata as Professor of Tropical Diseases. He also served the National Medical Institute, in charge of its Tropical Disease Ward. He was also the Head of the Department of Biochemistry and Honorary Professor of Biochemistry at the University College of Science, Calcutta.

Brahmachari played an important part in the formation of the world's second Blood Bank in Kolkata in 1939. He was the Chairman of the Blood Transfusion Service of Bengal. He was the Vice-President of the St. John Ambulance Association of the Bengal Branch and also its President. He was the first Indian to become the Chairman of the Managing Body of the Indian Red Cross Society of the Bengal Branch.

For his achievements, he received many awards, including the Griffith Memorial Prize of the University of Calcutta, the Minto Medal by the Calcutta School of Tropical Medicine and Hygiene (1921) and the Sir William Jones Medal by the Asiatic Society of Bengal.

He was awarded the title of *Rai Bahadur* and awarded the Kaisar-i-Hind Gold Medal, 1st Class by the Governor General Lord Lytton (1924), In 1934, he was conferred a Knighthood by the British Government (1934).

Brahmachari was a nominee for the Nobel Prize in 1929 in the category of physiology and medicine.

The Kolkata Municipal Corporation renamed Loudon Street the Dr UN Brahmachari Street.

DWARKANATH KOTNIS

Dr Dwarkanath Kotnis was born in a lower middle class family on October 10, 1910 in Sholapur, Mumbai. A vivacious kid by nature, Dr Kotnis forever aspired to become a doctor. After completing his graduation in medicine from GS Medical College, Bombay, he went on to pursue his postgraduation internship. However, he shelved his postgraduation plans when he got the chance to join the medical aid mission to China. In 1937, the communist General Zhu De requested Jawaharlal Nehru to send Indian physicians to China during the Second Sino-Japanese War to help the soldiers. A medical team of five doctors, including Dr Kotnis was sent as the part of Indian Medical Mission Team in September 1938. After the war, all other doctors except Dr Kotnis, returned back to India. Dr Kotnis decided to stay back and serve at the military base. Kotnis made China his home and joined the Communist Party of China, in July 1942. He also worked as a lecturer for sometime in the military area at the Dr Bethune Hygiene School. He took over the post of the first president of the Bethune International Peace Hospital after

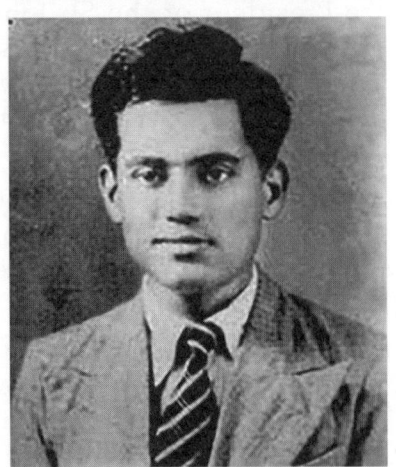

Dr Norman Bethune passed away. Due to inclement weather in China, inadequate diet, and enormous work strain, Dr Kotnis passed away following a sudden seizure attack in December 1942 at an early age of 32.

Dr Kotnis' major contribution was his selfless service to the Chinese soldiers in the battlefield during the Second Sino-Japanese War. He had the heart to stay back in China, even when his colleagues left, just for serving the wounded soldiers during the war. He was fondly dubbed as "Black Mother" by the Chinese villagers. Because of his loyalty, the young Indian doctor became a legendary figure in China and was honored by China with a gold medal during Sino-Japanese war of 1938, for saving thousands of Chinese lives. His role in solidifying relations between China and India has been humungous.

NAGARUR GOPINATH

Nagarur Gopinath (1922–2006) was born in Bellary, Karnataka. He passed the graduate degree in medicine from the Madras Medical College. He was one of the pioneers of open heart surgery and perfusion in India. He performed the first successful surgery for closure of an atrial and a ventricular septal defect at Christian Medical College and Hospital in 1962. He introduced pioneering methods in

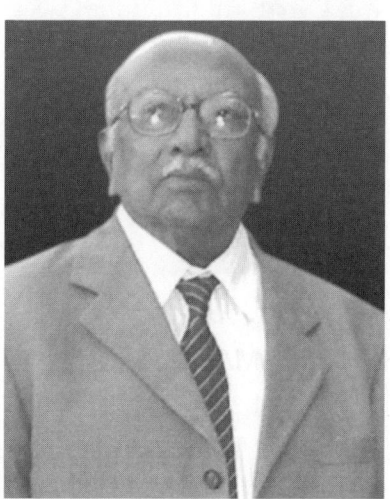

rheumatic heart surgery and cardiac pacemaker implantation in 1964. He established the department of cardiothoracic surgery AIIMS, New Delhi.

He was awarded the highest civilian honour of Padma Shri in 1974 by Government of India and Dr BC Roy Award, the highest Indian award in the medical category, from the Medical Council of India in 1978.

PROFULLA KUMAR SEN

(7th December 1915–22nd July 1982)

Indian vascular and cardiothoracic surgeon. He led the first human heart transplant procedure in India in 1968. Although the recipient died on the day of operation, he is credited to be the fourth surgeon in the world to carry out this operation. It was also the sixth attempt at this procedure in the world.

He was a talented poet and painter as well. His paintings were displayed once in the United States, and twice in India.

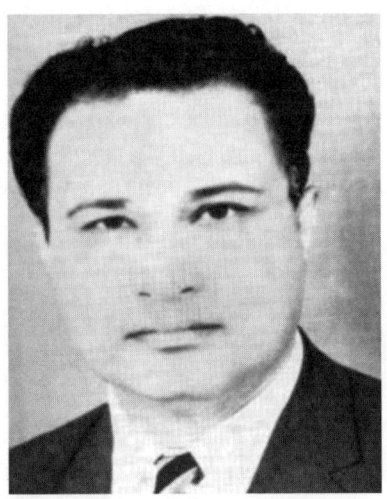

SAMBAMURTHY SUBRAMANIAN

(8th September 1933–17th July 2014)

Established international heart centre at Miami Children's Hospital. While at Buffalo Children's Hospital, he invented

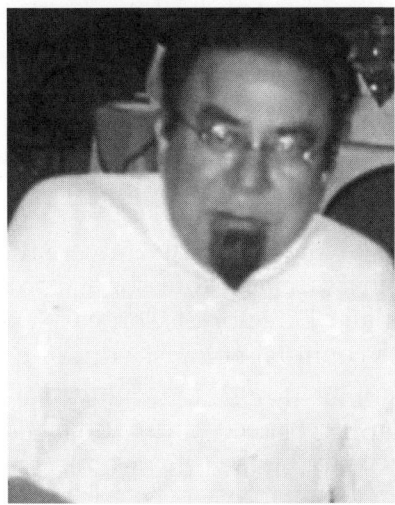

a surgical hypothermia chamber to perform relatively bloodless operations on infants.

RUSTOM JAL VAKIL

(17th July 1911–20th November 1974)

He was a cardiologist and pioneered the use of reserpine to control hypertension.

He was awarded Padma Bhushan award.

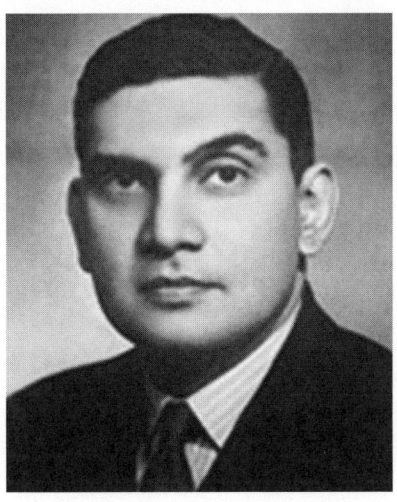

LIVING LEGENDS

BALAMURALI AMBATI

Dr Ambati was born in Vellore, Tamil Nadu, on July 29, 1977 and graduated from the Mount Sinai School of Medicine in New York city.

He is currently working in the Univeristy of Utah School of Medicine, is an Associate Professor of Ophthalmology and Visual Sciences and Director of Corneal Research. He is an Indian–American ophthalmologist, educator, and researcher.

He is known for being a child prodigy. He is the youngest doctor of the world, became a doctor at the age of 17. He also wrote a book on AIDS at the age of 11.

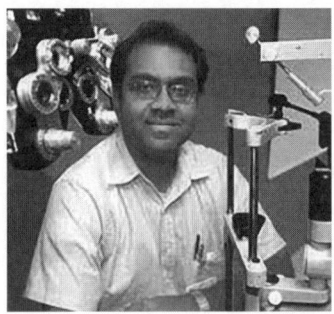

DEEPAK CHOPRA

Deepak Chopra is a renowned global personality who was born in New Delhi, India on October 22, 1946 and graduated

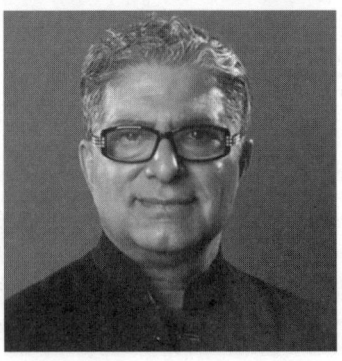

from All India Institute of Medical Sciences, New Delhi. He later on immigrated to America. Along with being a physician, he is a writer, who writes on Ayurveda and spirituality. He is also the founder of Chopra Foundation and is a public speaker. He has penned more than 57 books up until now.

DR DEVI PRASAD SHETTY

Dr Shetty was born at village Dakshina Kannada district, Karnataka, India on 8th May 1953. He graduated and after that postgraduated (in General Surgery) from Kasturba Medical College, Mangalore. He is a cardiac surgeon by profession and is called the Henry Ford (founder of the Ford Motor Company) of the heart surgery business for bringing change to the 'hearts' of India. He is the founder and also leads the world's largest and also the cheapest heart care institute called Narayana Hridayalaya.

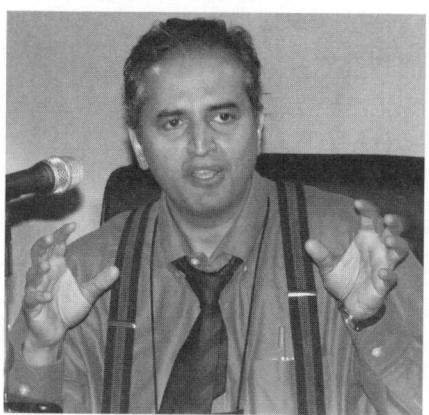

DR NARESH TREHAN

D Tehran was born on 12th August, 1946 at Batala, Punjab. He did his MBBS from KG Medical College, Lucknow (1968) and then went onto practice at New York University Medical Center Manhattan, USA.

He is a world renowned cardiovascular and cardiothoracic surgeon from India.

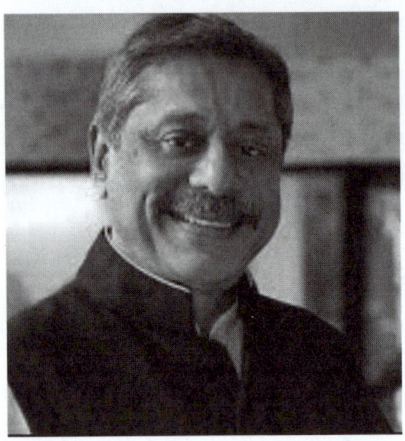

He has been serving as the Indian President's Personal Surgeon since 1991.

Apart from being honoured with many awards in the medicine field, Dr Trehan has also been the recipient of Padma Shri, Padma Bhushan and Lal Bahadur Shastri National Award.

He is currently the CEO and MD of Medanta, the Medicity.

DR SUNIL PRADHAN

Dr Pradhan was born on 25th June 1957 in Bijnor, Uttar Pradesh. He graduated (MBBS) in 1979 and postgraduated (MD) in Internal Medicine in 1983 from the King George's

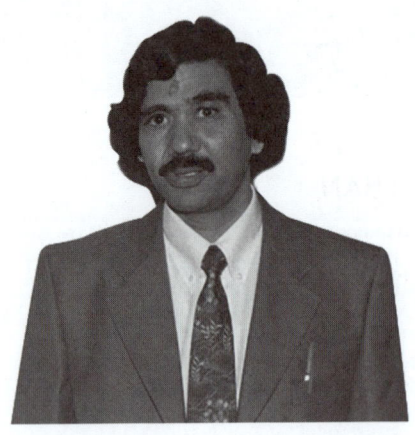

Medical University, Lucknow. He further pursued DM degree in neurology.

Dr Pradhan is a famous neurologist and medical researcher. He invented two electrophysiological techniques and contributed in describing five medical signs, one of which is now known as the Pradhan Sign.

His other researches are related to facioscapulohumeral muscular dystrophy (FSHD) and similar neuro diseases. Presently, he is working at Sanjay Gandhi Post Graduate Institute of Medical Sciences, Lucknow, UP.

He has been bestowed with Padma Shri and numerous other awards.

DR ASHOK RAJGOPAL

Dr Rajgopal was born on 30th September 1953, in Bengaluru, Karnataka. He obtained MBBS degree from Armed Forces Medical College, Pune in 1974 and MS degree from All India Institute of Medical Sciences, New Delhi, in 1978. He went onto obtain MCH degree from University of Liverpool. He is also a Fellow of International Medical Sciences Academy, FIMSA (1996) and a Fellow of the Royal College of Surgeons of Edinburgh (2010).

Dr Ashok Rajgopal is India's wonder man in the field of orthopaedic surgery having more than 20,000 arthroscopic and over 28,000 arthroplasty surgeries successfully.

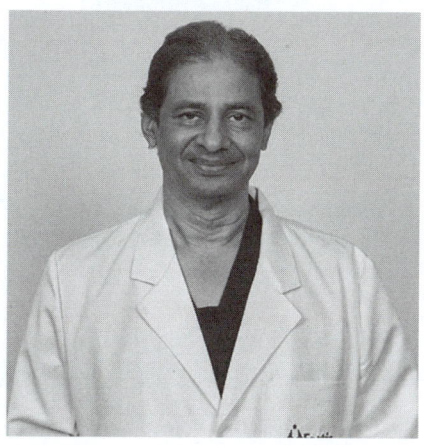

He became the first Orthopaedic Surgeon in India, to perform a virtual total knee replacement surgery and contributed to the development of the latest knee implant—Persona Knee System.

He was honored with Padma Shri in 2014.

Presently, he is acting as Chairman of Medanta Bone and Joint Institute and head of knee division at Medanta—The Medicity, Gurugram.

DR SUNDARAM NATARAJAN

Hailing from a family of ophthalmologists, Dr Sundaram Natarajan is a leading specialist in medical and surgical eye problems. He laid foundation Aditya Jyot Eye Hospital, Mumbai, in 1990 and presently works as its chief managing director.

In 2005, Dr APJ Abdul Kalam (former President of India) visited this hospital and expressed his desire to put a twinkle in the eyes of the visually impaired. Following which not-for-profit body, Aditya Jyot Foundation for Twinkling Little Eyes (AJFTLE) was established. AJFTLE works with a mission to alleviate the suffering of the poor, neglected population and aims to prevent avoidable blindness through

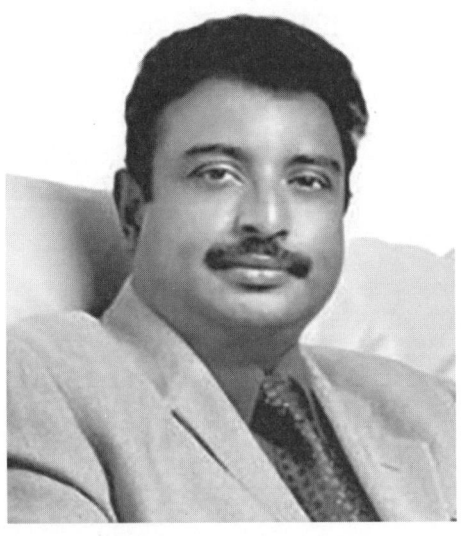

awareness generation, eye screening and providing access to quality eye care at an affordable cost. The foundation runs outreach programs in rural and urban slums and tribal areas that strive to provide quality eye care for the underprivileged. The organization takes special interest in promoting eye donation.

For his accomplishments in the field of medicine, he was conferred with Padma Shri in 2013.

BELLE MONAPPA HEGDE

Belle Monappa Hegde, often abbreviated as **BM Hegde** was born 18th August 1938 in Pangala, Udupi, Karnataka. He is an eminent cardiologist, professional educator and an author.

Dr Hegde obtained MBBS degree from Stanley Medical College (Madras) and MD from King George Medical College (Lucknow), FRCP from Royal College of Physicians, London, Glasgow, Edinburgh, and Dublin. He also received training in cardiology from Harvard Medical School.

Formerly he has acted as Vice Chancellor of Manipal University, as co-chairman of the TAG-VHS Diabetes Research Centre, Chennai and as chairman of Bharatiya Vidya Bhavan, Mangalore. He has authored several books on medical practice and ethics. He is also the Editor in Chief of the medical journal, *Journal of the Science of Healing Outcomes*. He was awarded the Dr BC Roy Award in 1999 and Padma Bhushan in 2010.

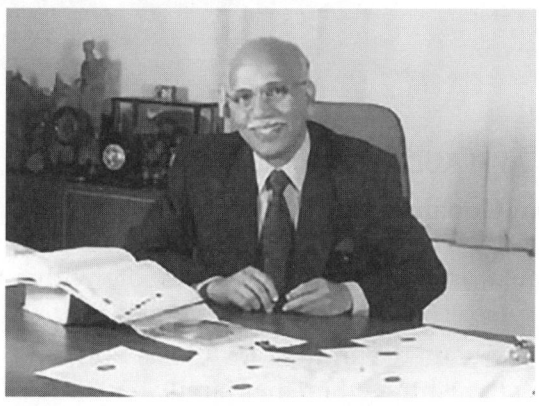

ABHAY BANG AND RANI BANG

The Bangs are honored for their leadership in community-based health care. They are Indian social activists and researchers working in the Gadchiroli district of Maharashtra, India. The programme designed by them has substantially reduced infant mortality rates in one of the most poverty-stricken areas in the world. The WHO and UNICEF have endorsed their approach to treating newborn babies and the programme is currently being rolled out across India and in parts of Africa.

The Bangs founded the Society for Education, Action and Research in Community Health (SEARCH)—a non-profit organisation, which is involved in rural health service and research.

The couple has been awarded the Maharashtra Bhushan Award.

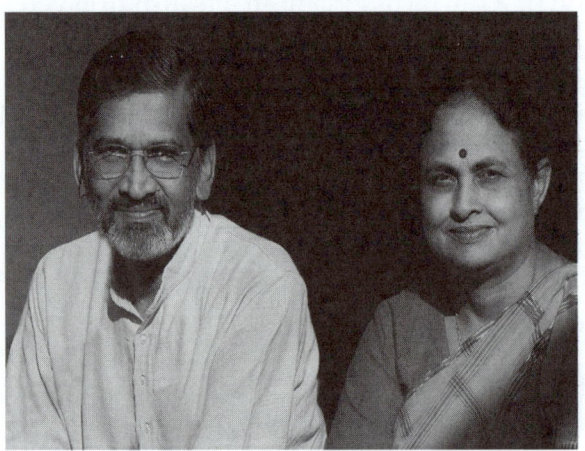

WOMEN APPLAUDABE AS DOCTORS

Anandibai Gopalrao Joshi (31st March 1865–26th February 1887) was the first woman from the erstwhile Bombay presidency of India to study and graduate with a two-year degree in western medicine in the United States.

Originally named Yamuna, Joshi was born and raised in Kalyan, Maharashtra, where her family had previously been landlords before experiencing financial losses. As per the practice at that time she was married at the age of nine to Gopalrao Joshi, a widower almost 20 years older than her. After marriage, Yamuna's husband renamed her 'Anandi'. Gopalrao Joshi worked as a postal clerk in Kalyan and later transferred to Kolkata (Calcutta). He was the man to encourage her study medicine. He was so obsessed with his wife's education that he would abuse and beat her. So much so that one day when he found her cooking in kitchen he went into fits of rage. At the age of 14, Anandibai gave birth to a boy, but the child lived only for 10 days for lack of medical care. This proved to be a turning point in Anandi's life and inspired her to become a physician.

In 1880, Gopalrao sent a letter to Royal Wilder, a well-known American missionary, stating his wife's interest in studying medicine in the United States and inquiring about a suitable post in the US for himself. Wilder published the correspondence in his Princeton's Missionary Review. Theodicia Carpenter, a resident of Roselle, New Jersey, happened to read it while waiting to see her dentist. Impressed by both Anandibai's desire to study medicine, and Gopalrao's support for his wife, she wrote to Anandibai. Carpenter and Anandibai developed a close friendship and came to refer to each other as "aunt" and "niece". Later, Carpenter hosted Anandibai in Rochelle during her stay in the US.

On learning of Joshis' plans to pursue higher education in the west, orthodox Indian society opposed them very strongly. Anandibai addressed the community at Serampore College Hall, in West Bengal, explaining her decision to go to America and obtain a medical degree. She discussed the hostility and ill-treatment, she and her husband were facing. She stressed the need for female doctors in India, emphasizing that Hindu women could better serve as physicians to Hindu women. Her speech received publicity, and financial contributions started pouring in from all over India.

Anandibai travelled to New York from Kolkata (Calcutta) by ship. In New York, Theodicia Carpenter received her in

June 1883. Anandibai got herself enrolled in Woman's Medical College of Pennsylvania (Fig. 25).

Anandibai began her medical training at age of 19. While she was in India, she had suffered from weakness, constant headaches, occasional fever, and sometimes breathlessness. In America, her health worsened because of the cold weather and unfamiliar diet. She contracted tuberculosis. Nevertheless, she graduated with an MD in March of 1886. The topic of her thesis was "Obstetrics among the Aryan Hindoos." On her graduation, Queen Victoria sent her a congratulatory message.

In late 1886, Anandibai returned to India, receiving a grand welcome. The princely state of Kolhapur appointed her as

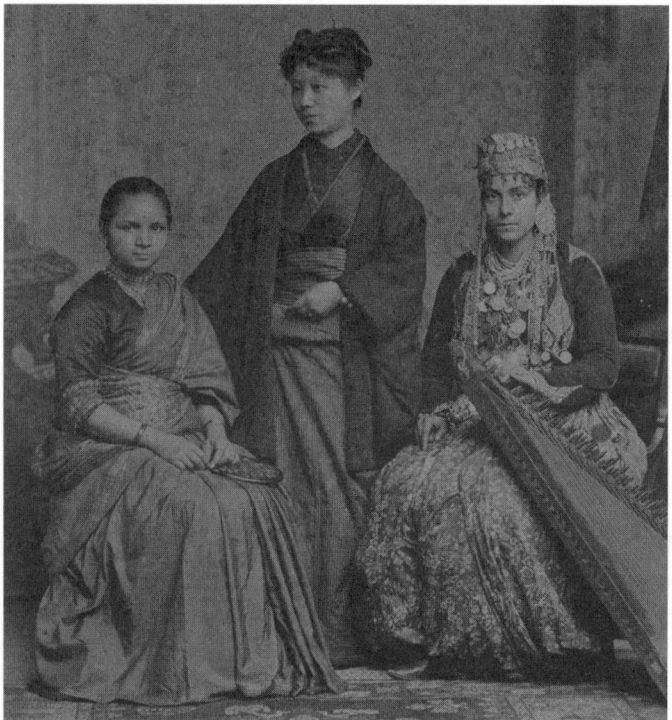

Fig. 25: Woman's Medical College of Pennsylvania in 1886. Anandibai Joshi, from India (left) with Kei Okami, Japan (center) and Sabat Islambooly, from Syria (right). All three completed their medical studies and each of them was the first woman from their respective countries to obtain a degree in western medicine

the physician-in-charge of the female ward of the local Albert Edward Hospital.

Anandibai died of tuberculosis early the next year on 26th February 1887 before turning 22. Her death was mourned throughout India. Her ashes were sent to Theodicia Carpenter, who placed them in her family cemetery with inscription stating that Anandi Joshi was a Hindu Brahmin girl, the first Indian woman to receive education abroad and to obtain a medical degree.

KADAMBANI GANGULY

Kadambani was born in a liberal family during the British Raj on 18th July 1861 at Bhagalpur, Bihar.

She studied medicine at the Calcutta Medical College and was awarded graduate degree in 1886. At that she became one of the two Indian women doctors who qualified to practice western medicine, Anandi Gopal Joshi being the other. (One more Indian woman by the name of Abala Bose passed entrance in 1881 but was refused admission to the medical college and went to Madras to study medicine but never graduated!)

Battling stereotypes and refusing to fall into the norm of marriage, and family-rearing Ganguly travelled overseas to

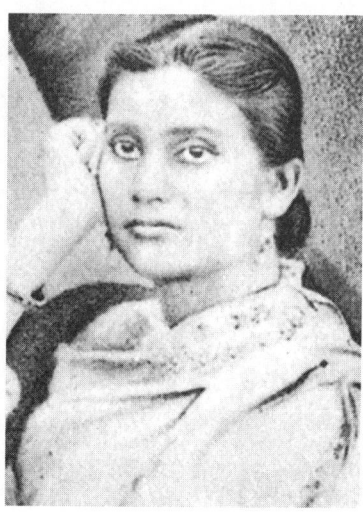

the UK, and returned home only after she had LRCP, LRCS, and GFPS degrees attached to her name. Garnering a better reputation among her male counterparts and superiors, she was offered a job with Lady Dufferin Hospital, Kolkata, following which she began her own practice. Her work was the stepping stone for women aspiring for a career in medicine and was responsible for the countless numbers she inspired to join in the same.

DR SIVARAMAKRISHNA IYER PADMAVATI

Dr Sivaramakrishna Iyer Padmavati is the first female Cardiologist of India.

She was born on 20th June 1917 at Myanmar, Burma. She studied her MBBS at Rangoon Medical Collegeand then moved to London in 1949, where she received an FRCP from the Royal College of Physicians, London, followed by an FRCPE from the Royal College of Physicians, Edinburgh. She started practising medicine in a number of famous hospitals in London before she developed interest in cardiology. Studying further into the subject, she realized that cardiology in India did not receive the importance it was due. Returning to her homeland, she had successfully set up the country's first cardiology clinic and also created the first cardiology department in an Indian medical college.

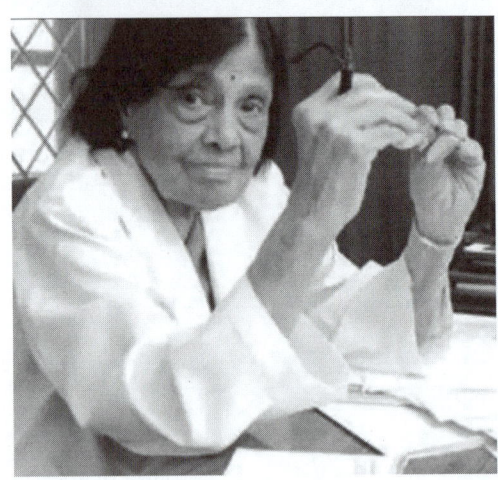

A recipient of the Padma Vibhushan (1992), Padmavati has acted as the director of the National Heart Institute, Delhi, and the Founder President of the All India Heart Foundation. Besides this, she also collaborates with the World Health Organisation in training students in preventive cardiology.

INDIRA HINDUJA

Dr Indira Hinduja will always be remembered for delivering the country's first test-tube baby, all the way back in 1986. A gynaecologist, obstetrician, and infertility specialist, she received her medical degree from Mumbai University and has been practicing in her hometown since. Hinduja is also credited with inventing the Gamete intrafallopian transfer (GIFT) technique, which resulted in the birth of the country's first GIFT baby in 1988. Practicing in PD Hinduja National Hospital and Medical Research Centre, she is also associated with developing an oocyte donation technique for menopausal and premature ovarian failure patients.

She was awarded the prestigious Padma Shri by the Government in 2011.

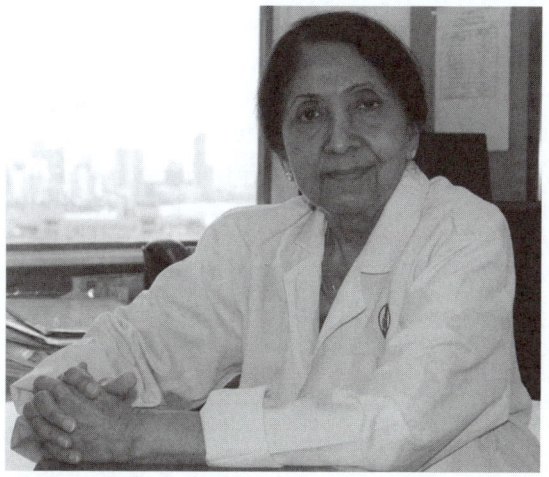

KAMINI RAO

Considering the state of health-care in South India even a few years ago, Dr Kamini Rao's contributions to fertility and

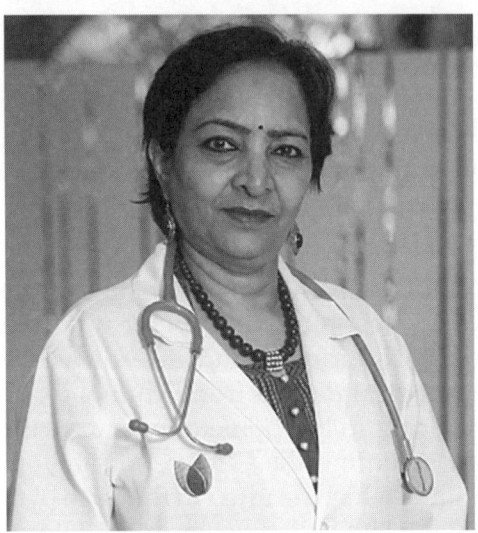

reproductive endocrinology is no small feat. She spent her early life at Bangluru and studied at St John's Medical College. Thereafter, afer spending several years in professional training and practice in the UK, Rao returned to South India with advanced knowledge in gynaecology and is credited with the birth of India's first SIFT (transvaginal sperm intra-fallopian transfer) baby. Along with this, she also set up South India's first Semen Bank and also engineered its first babies born through ICSI (intra cytoplasmic sperm injection) and Laser Assisted Hatching.

For all her contributions to Indian medicine, particularly in introducing new and innovative fertility measures, she was awarded the Padma Shri in 2014.

DR NEELAM KLER

Neelam Kler was born in Srinagar, Jammu and Kashmir, in India. She obtained her MBBS and then MD in Pediatrics from the Post-Graduate Institute of Medical Sciences and Research (PIGMER), Chandigarh, and continued there for further training in neonatology. Later, she went to Copenhagen, Denmark, on a fellowship in neonatology from the Copenhagen University for advanced studies on the subject.

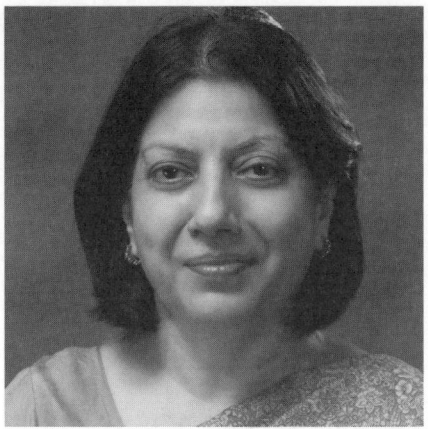

She started her professional career in India by joining department of neonatology at Sir Ganga Ram Hospital, New Delhi, in 1988. Presently, she holds the position of the Chairperson there.

Dr Kler has proved her mettle in neonatology, a subspecialty of paediatrics with her innovative and pioneering work in the field of neonatal intensive care and ventilation.

She had developed neonatal care to improve the survival rate of extremely tiny preterm babies (less than 1000 grams) to 90%.

For this, she was awarded the Padma Bhushan in 2014.

The number of achievers in field of medicine from India is countless. Few names that I have written about are sufficient to spark interest in my students to gather knowledge about as many others as they can. Best wishes for many more achievers!

Ongoing Journey

The preceding chapters undoubtedly prove that history of medicine is endlessly fascinating. It gives an insight as to how early civilizations coped with health problems. This information contributes to our present understanding of medicine and healing.

Every human civilization developed a system of medicine, based on material medica, spells, incantations, magic and rituals. Each has progressed from primitive stage to a regular system of medicine. To maintain good health, cure diseases, and to care for wounds and broken bones was as important to our ancestors as it is to us today and every civilization made best endeavors to keep its population healthy. Over the times, as the human civilizations advanced, the disease pattern changed and so changed the pattern of practice of medicine.

We shall free medicine from its worst errors. Not by following that which those of old taught, but by our own observation of nature, confirmed by extensive practice and long experience.

—Paracelsus, 1530

Very aptly said by Paracelsus. Learning from history, today doctors stress on healthy living, prevention of disease, personal and social hygiene and not merely the cure of diseases. Moreover as a result of globalization, today we are exposed to various patterns of medicine and are in beneficial situation of availing best from each pattern of medicine.

I had started this enthralling saga of man's struggle against disease from prehistoric times and waded out of the history to doctors presently creating history from our own country.

Now at this point I wish to pause. I leave it entirely to my readers to dive into ocean of history to depths in accordance to their individual level of inquisitiveness.

Further Reading

Following is a list of relevant books which can be referred to for further reading.

1. A Brief History of Medicine: From Hippocrates to Gene Therapy (Brief Histories) by Paul Strathern, Robinson publisher.
2. A Concise History of Medicine by Osler William(1919), Kesinger Publication.
3. A History of Medicine by Lois N Magner, Taylor and Francis Group publishers.
4. A History of Medicine: I. Primitive and Archaic Medicine by Henry Ernst Sigerist, Oxford University Press Inc publishers.
5. A History of Medicine: II. Early Greek, Hindu, and Persian Medicine by Henry Ernst Sigerist, Oxford University Press Inc publishers.
6. Ancient Medicine (Sciences of Antiquity) by Vivian Nutton, Routledge publisher.
7. Disease, Medicine and Society in England, 1550-1860 (New Studies in Economic and Social History) by Roy Porter, Cambridge University Press.
8. Greatest Benefit To Mankind: A Medical History Of Humanity (The Norton History of Science) by Roy Porter, WW Norton publisher.
9. History of Medicine by RK Marya, Jaypee Brothers Medical Publishers.
10. History of Medicine from the Earliest Ages to the Commencement of the Nineteenth Century by Robley Dunglison, Nabu Press.
11. History of Medicine in 100 facts by Caroline Rance, Amberley Publishing.
12. Medicine Across Cultures: History and Practice of Medicine in Non-Western Cultures (Science Across

Cultures: The History of Non-Western Science) by Helaine Selin, Kluwer Academic Publishers.

13. Medieval and Early Renaissance Medicine by Siraisi, University of Chicago Press.

14. Medieval Islamic Medicine (The New Edinburgh Islamic Surveys) by Peter E. Pormann, Edinburgh University Press.

15. Revolutionary Medicine (Illustrated Living History Series) by C Keith Wilbur, Globe Pequot Press.

16. Science and the Practice of Medicine in the Nineteenth Century (Cambridge Studies in the History of Science) by WF Bynum, Cambridge University Press.

17. The Beginnings of Western Science by Lindberg, University of Chicago Press.

18. The Cambridge History of Medicine by Roy Porter, Cambridge University Press.

19. The Doctor's Oath: An Essay in the History of Medicine by WHS Jones, Cambridge University Press.

20. The Western Medical Tradition: 800 BC to AD 1800 by Lawrence I. Conrad, Cambridge University Press.

Index

Reader's Notes

Reader's Notes

Reader's Notes

Reader's Notes